Hans-Rudolf Weiss

I Have Scoliosis

A Guidebook for Patients, Family Members, and Therapists

Hans-Rudolf Weiss

Impressum / Imprint
Bibliografische Information der Deutschen Nationalbibliothek: Die Deutsche Nationalbibliothek verzeichnet diese Publikation in der Deutschen Nationalbibliografie; detaillierte bibliografische Daten sind im Internet über http://dnb.d-nb.de abrufbar.
Alle in diesem Buch genannten Marken und Produktnamen unterliegen warenzeichen-, marken- oder patentrechtlichem Schutz bzw. sind Warenzeichen oder eingetragene Warenzeichen der jeweiligen Inhaber. Die Wiedergabe von Marken, Produktnamen, Gebrauchsnamen, Handelsnamen, Warenbezeichnungen u.s.w. in diesem Werk berechtigt auch ohne besondere Kennzeichnung nicht zu der Annahme, dass solche Namen im Sinne der Warenzeichen- und Markenschutzgesetzgebung als frei zu betrachten wären und daher von jedermann benutzt werden dürften.

Bibliographic information published by the Deutsche Nationalbibliothek: The Deutsche Nationalbibliothek lists this publication in the Deutsche Nationalbibliografie; detailed bibliographic data are available in the Internet at http://dnb.d-nb.de.
Any brand names and product names mentioned in this book are subject to trademark, brand or patent protection and are trademarks or registered trademarks of their respective holders. The use of brand names, product names, common names, trade names, product descriptions etc. even without a particular marking in this work is in no way to be construed to mean that such names may be regarded as unrestricted in respect of trademark and brand protection legislation and could thus be used by anyone.

Coverbild / Cover image: www.ingimage.com

Verlag / Publisher:
LAP LAMBERT Academic Publishing
ist ein Imprint der / is a trademark of
OmniScriptum GmbH & Co. KG
Bahnhofstraße 28, 66111 Saarbrücken, Deutschland / Germany
Email: info@omniscriptum.com

Herstellung: siehe letzte Seite /
Printed at: see last page
ISBN: 978-3-659-49541-0

Copyright © Hans-Rudolf Weiss
Copyright © 2013 OmniScriptum GmbH & Co. KG
Alle Rechte vorbehalten. / All rights reserved. Saarbrücken 2013

Dr. med. Hans-Rudolf Weiss

I Have Scoliosis

A Guidebook for Patients, Family Members, and Therapists

10th revised edition

Contents:

Preface 5

Foreword to the 10th edition 7

1 Introduction 11

2 Patient Reports 15
    Scoliosis Report No. 1 16
    Scoliosis Report No. 2 20
    Scoliosis Report No. 3 22
    Scoliosis Report No. 4 23
    Scoliosis Report No. 5 25
    Scoliosis Report No. 6 27
    Scoliosis Report No. 7 30
    Scoliosis Report No. 8 33
    Scoliosis Report No. 9 35
    Scoliosis Report No. 10 36
    Scoliosis Report No. 11 38
    Scoliosis Report No. 12 40
    Scoliosis Report No. 13 41

3 Scoliosis – What's That? 45
    3.1 The Course of Untreated Idiopathic Scoliosis 46
    3.2 The Course of Treated Idiopathic Scoliosis 47

4 What Has to Be Measured? 51
    4.1 Radiography 51
    4.2 Clinical Measuring Procedures 57
    4.3 Surface Topography 58

5 Treatment 63
    5.1 Physical Rehabilitation 63
    5.2 Brace Treatment 69
        5.2.1 Design Variants of Trunk Orthoses in Scoliosis Therapy 77
        5.2.2 Learning to Wear a Brace 85
        5.2.3 Treatment Duration and Weaning off the Brace 87

  5.2.4 Frequently Asked Questions (FAQ) – What Can Patients Expect from Bracing?.. 89
  5.2.5 Future Developments in Brace Treatment – a Perspective 100
 5.3 Operation and Surgical Procedures 102
  5.3.1 Posterior Access 104
  5.3.2 Anterior Access..104
  5.3.3 Current State of Development of Instruments Used for Scoliosis Correction.. 106

6 What Restrictions Do I Have to Expect 113
 6.1 Scoliosis and Sports 113
 6.2 Scoliosis and Pregnancy..114
 6.3 Scoliosis and Osteoporosis 115
 6.4 What Do I Have to Expect in Old Age?...117
  6.4.1 Pain 117
  6.4.2 Cardiovascular Problems...117
 6.5 Scoliosis and the Psyche 118

7 Guidelines: Indication for Treating Cases of Scoliosis (status 6 / 2013)... 121

8 Summary.. 129

Conservative specialists... 131

Annex: Instructions for Use.. 137

Literature 145

Preface (for the 9th edition)

For three generations now, our family has had a vocational and personal calling to treat scoliosis. My mother, Katharina Schroth, developed what she called the "three-dimensional scoliosis treatment" before 1920. As a child, I was already involved with the treatment of scoliosis patients, and in the end I decided to pursue a career as a physical therapist. In Sobernheim in 1961, together with my mother, I established an institute for rehabilitating patients with spinal deformities, where, under my direction, up to 150 patients were housed and treated according to our intense treatment concept. In the 1980s, my son Dr. med. Hans-Rudolf Weiss teamed up with his wife to develop a Germany-wide advanced training program for physiotherapists. Thanks to his scientific work as the head physician of what was then the Katharina Schroth Clinic, the effectiveness of our method was able to be demonstrated. Since that time, the three-dimensional scoliosis treatment according to Katharina Schroth has caught on around the world.

Up until the 1970s, my mother and I almost exclusively treated patients with very severe scoliosis. At the end of the 1970s, it finally occurred to me that there are different curvature patterns, each of which requires its own method of treatment. In addition, my son's findings are the basis for treating more mild curvatures differently than pronounced ones, a concept with successful results. Even treatment using braces has become simpler nowadays. As late as in the 1980s, around 50 percent of scoliosis victims could not wear their braces due to pain. The devices were quite large, sometimes reaching all the way from the thighs to the chin (Milwaukee brace). Even the brace developed by Dr. Chêneau from Toulouse originally protruded a fair amount, causing adverse effects beyond merely cosmetic considerations. In 1999, my son was the first to develop a better Chêneau brace. Since then, it has become clear that one pelvic half of the brace can generally be done without and that, for some curvature patterns, even a short design delivers excellent results. For those who are afflicted, the developments that have taken place in our family's history have been a true blessing. According to the current state of knowledge, the prospect of success offered by non-surgical scoliosis treatment is greater than 95 percent. The physiotherapeutic treatment has been simplified and the braces relatively comfortable to wear and no longer causing major discomfort, provided that treatment is being monitored by an experienced physician.

I am happy and proud that my son has been so successful in taking up this traditional pursuit of our family and that the developmental process initiated on behalf of the patients continues on. This guidebook, which is now being published in its 9th edition, has already been a great help to many scoliosis patients. Especially at a time when a great many contradicting and dubious things are being spread over the Internet, scientifically verified information from the pen of an expert is extremely valuable. That is why I hope this book enjoys a wide circulation.

Bad Sobernheim, early 2013

Christa Lehnert-Schroth

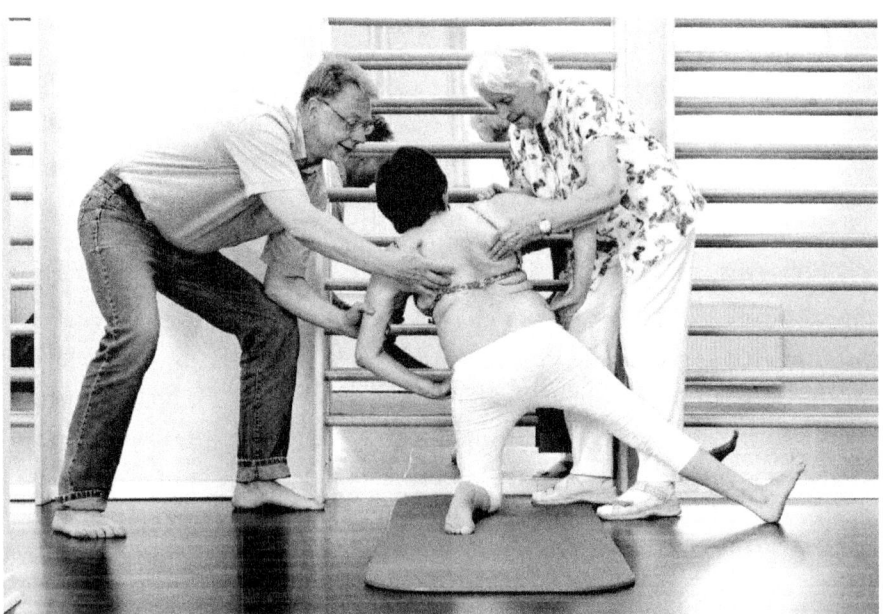

Christa Lehnert-Schroth and her son Dr. Hans-Rudolf Weiss treating a patient

Foreword to the 10th edition

Even though the 9th edition was still relatively current, there have been a few more new and recent discoveries that I do not wish to withhold from my readers. For this reason, I have done the usual updating of this 10th edition of my scoliosis guidebook and have slightly expanded it.

In the meantime, there have been independent studies backing up the current developments in the field of physiotherapy.

By studying the current specialist literature, more and more evidence can be found for the effectiveness of physiotherapeutic treatment. And even treatment with a brace can now be regarded as having a scientific basis. Meanwhile there is evidence for brace treatment (one randomized controlled study) and for correcting exercises (four randomized controlled studies) on the highest level (level I). In contrast to that, an ever greater number of current studies on long-term results make it clear that there is no evidence for the effectiveness of surgical scoliosis treatment. In fact, it has been demonstrated with increasing frequency that a scoliosis operation leads to greater long-term complications than if the condition had been left untreated. Despite these disturbing facts, the potential long-term complications are usually not discussed in scientific publications.

Even though a scoliosis operation today should be done with great care and require that the patient be fully informed – particularly with respect to long-term complications – I have included the chapter on surgical scoliosis treatment more or less unchanged. For there may be some patients who indeed decide to go with an operation. Nevertheless, it is important to realize that the operation results that this book testifies to are not able to be achieved at just any surgical facility.

The future, however, belongs to the conservative (non-surgical) treatment of scoliosis. It is certainly a relief for patients to hear that the newest developments offer a greater than 90 percent chance of preventing the curvature from increasing or of considerably reducing the angle of curvature for cases where the angle of curvature is between 20 and 50 degrees. This is accomplished by a brace and physiotherapy and possibly even inpatient rehabilitation, all working together. The newest strategies in physiotherapy aim for results that are acceptable for everyday living and affect the afflicted persons as little as possible. This follows the motto "Do exercises so that you will no longer have to" and not "Do the exercises just for the sake of doing them." After only a short time and without any major theoretical training, a sense of postural awareness can be engendered safely and properly that helps to avoid the day-to-day curvature-stimulating behavior.

Bracing today has largely been improved. Computer aided design (CAD) and computer aided manufacturing (CAM) allows to standardize brace treatment. On this basis the Gensingen brace (CBW) has been developed with a brace library which is most comfortable and highly effective. Meanwhile this series of CAD braces worldwide is the most common CAD series today.

Adult patients with scoliosis usually have no pains. But if there are signs and symtoms in an adult they should seek individual advice from a conservative specialist in this field. Updated conservative specialists can be found here: https://schrothbestpractice.com/physical-rehabilitation-schroth-best-practice-standard/.

I wish to thank all the patients having supported this book with their contributions, with their stories and with their pictures, especially Andra, Kristina, Sanne and Tiyen!

This book has been translatet to English by Cambridge Editing and I am thankful for the excellent and timely service!

My dear friend, Kathryn Moramarco finally has gone over the manuscript and has sorted out the last mistakes. I appreciate your constant help so much!

Finally, I wish to thank Vitalie Rotaru, Lambert Academic Publishing, for his outstanding efforts and great support for the final production process of this book.

Gensingen in Summer 2016

Dr. med. Hans-Rudolf Weiss

Dedicated to all my courageous scoliosis patients

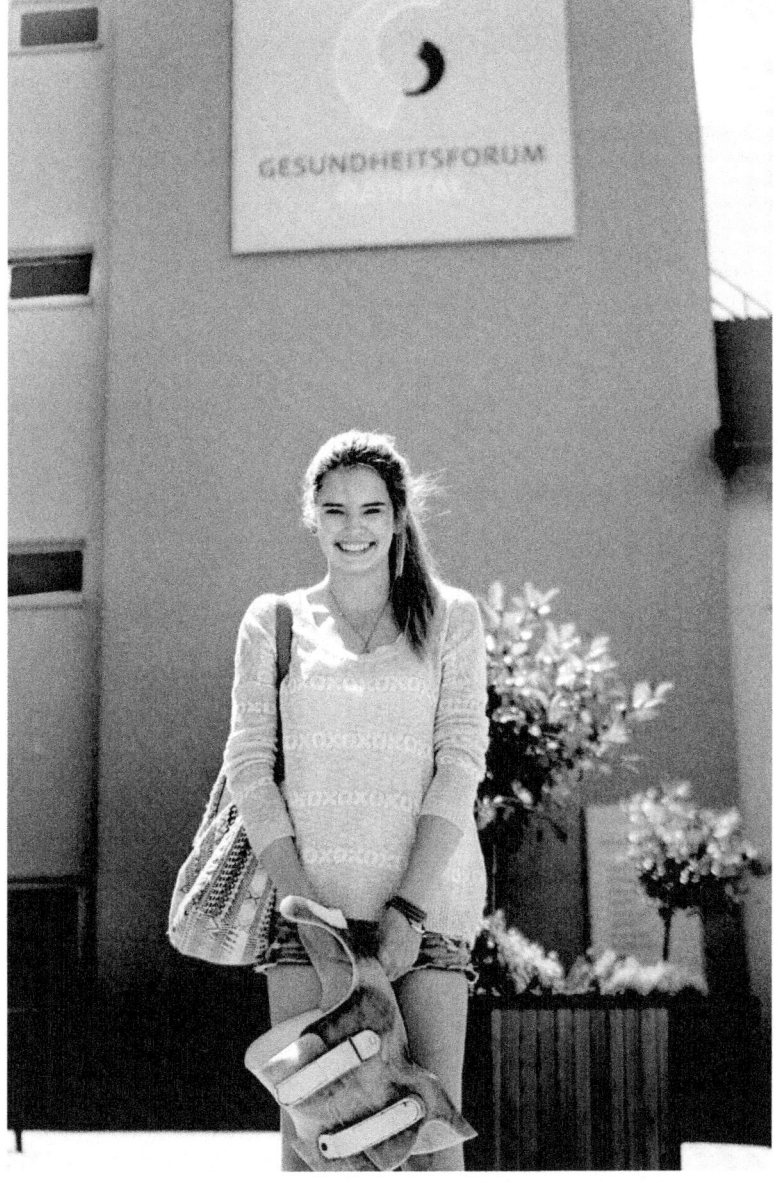

1 Introduction

How do children, adolescents, and parents of those afflicted receive the diagnosis of "scoliosis"?

Some register the diagnosis and go back to everyday life without giving the consequences of this diagnosis much thought. While others are broadsided by the diagnosis as if it were a death sentence. Despair and deep depressions are often the result.

And yet there is nothing bad about scoliosis in and of itself. Viewed from a medical standpoint, it is usually just a growth disturbance in a child or adolescent who, as a rule, is otherwise healthy and capable.

The thing that evidently makes scoliosis so terrible for the one person and causes the other to suppress the diagnosis is the varied and conflicting information, some of it overly dramatized, that is associated with the diagnosis.

People say: "If scoliosis is not treated, you will eventually have to use a wheelchair." Or, "If the curvature is not treated right, you will be sure to have back pain." Other things people say include: "In adult years, the curvature will get worse and worse and will eventually snap," or even, "With a deformity like that in the area of the ribcage, the curvature presses against the heart, causing you to die sooner."

Such views would cause any of us to be utterly dejected. But they cannot be reasoned away, even though – from a scientific point of view – most of them are untrue.

In order to keep treatment strategies for scoliosis in perspective, and increase a patient's chances for success, I decided to write this guidebook starting with the first German edition in 1999. From a medical standpoint, scoliosis by itself need not lead to wild conclusions. Still, it is true some of the successful treatment strategies are rather involved and can adversely affect the quality of life in certain stages of life.

After all, who wants to do physical therapy every day; who wants to wear a brace for 23 hours a day for years on end; and, most of all, who wants to undergo an operation to stiffen the spinal column? To be sure, involved treatment measures can only be carried out after providing more detailed information, which can often be viewed as vexing.

Is it not a bitter pill to swallow for the afflicted person that wearing a brace has a high chance of success at the very time when the sex drive of the young patient is coming into bloom? "Now that I've found a boy who's really cute, I have to wear a brace. Isn't that a handicap?" Indeed, this can be a social handicap and have a damaging effect on dating. Very few cases of scoliosis lead to severe physical impairment, but a social handicap could be a very serious thing, especially when it comes at a time that is very important for adolescents.

There is another thing that this booklet is meant to highlight: Not every method of treatment is right for everyone. For instance, there are patients who reject the brace. If this refusal persists despite detailed information from a competent orthopedist, I rule out the possibility of successful results from using a brace.

Also, an operation is not the right thing for many people. If anxieties about an operation cannot be defused even by extensive explanations from the surgeon, then this kind of an operation is certainly not the right plan of action.

It is also possible that neither a brace nor an operation nor even intensive physical therapy appear to be doable. In such cases, guiding and attending the afflicted person is very challenging. Perhaps the doctor simply has to wait and see how the scoliosis plays out without treatment.

A scoliosis specialist should accompany the patient on his/her journey and suggest possible treatments. Even if the doctor is fully convinced of the merits of certain methods of treatment, trying to exert pressure on the afflicted person often has the opposite effect. In other words, it can tend to prevent the patient from accepting the treatment measures. For this reason, I see it as my responsibility to provide advice and explanations. Before patients can come to a decision, they have to understand all of the different vantage points and recognize the consequences their decision might have. Only then can they choose the right path, embark on the trail to successful treatment, and follow it through.

I keep hearing the same thing from certain colleagues: "A scoliosis physician has to be a strict doctor!" I do not share this opinion. If I am too strict with my patients as their doctor, this can have an adverse effect on the level of trust in the relationship. The result is that my patients will no longer tell me that they do not actually wear the brace. It is only by warmth and openness in the doctor-patient relationship that it is possible to recognize early on when obstacles to treatment are setting in. If an early onset of physical growth is "wreaking havoc" on my task as the treating physician, I simply have to go ahead and have a discussion with the patient sooner than I had planned about the potential consequences of wearing a brace for too short a time. I can still see in my mind the slide of a little girl in a swimming suit and a brace under a sunshade at the beach, which a colleague showed at a presentation he gave concerning the brace treatment of this girl's scoliosis, saying that the brace had to be worn in every case and under all circumstances for 23 hours a day.

I am extremely troubled by that. Of course it has to be stressed how important it is to wear braces for 23 hours a day during the primary growth spurt, since they are otherwise ineffective. When this is truly adhered to, then it is possible to make the occasional exception as a reward. So then, is it really a big problem if the brace is not worn to the disco on Saturday evenings for four to five hours? Is it really a big problem if the brace is only worn for 12 to 16 hours a day for 14 days during summer vacation, when it is otherwise worn for 23 hours a day the rest of the year? Is it really such a big problem if the brace is not worn but half the day on a week-long ski holiday?

I do not believe so. It is much easier to motivate the patient to accept such an involved treatment regimen of wearing a brace plus physical therapy if the joie de vivre can be experienced without the brace from time to time.

It should be pointed out that regularly wearing it for only half the day is not enough. However, if the brace is worn consistently on 300 days of the year, with four hours of wearing time missed only now and again, then any negative effects on the overall progress will be negligible.

Quite the contrary, the prospect of being allowed to take off the brace on special occasions will perk up an afflicted person's zest for life to such a degree that this may well have a psychologically reinforcing effect on straightening the posture.

Having the patient be responsible for following through on his/her own treatment promises the best possible success. If parents have to tell their child every single day: "You still have to do your exercises!" or "Now you've already had your brace off for yet another eight hours!" then the treatment will be less favorable. If puberty-related conflicts and the power struggle within the family is transferred to scoliosis treatment, it will not be blessed with success. For this reason, this is another topic that has to be brought up with the parents and child. The key questions are, "How much support does my child need?" or "Do I trust that my child can manage his responsibility on his own?"

If by saying yes to the final question the parents can signal to their child that they trust him/her, this very trust is what will most likely be rewarded with successful treatment.

Going back to the opening point of my introduction then, neither suppressing nor dramatizing scoliosis is the right way to go. It is my right as the afflicted person to be sad and angry; I have the right to cry and express my feelings. I can tell those around me that it hurts me to have scoliosis and that I am afraid of going through an involved regimen of treatment. Once these initial feelings have subsided, however, the second part of processing all this needs to occur, namely that of overcoming scoliosis. The degree to which I accept the scoliosis as "my scoliosis" and personally decide to pursue a treatment that promises success will in turn be the measure of how successful and persistent I am with regard to the treatment, since I will have been responsible for following it through myself.

The methods and coping mechanisms of each of my patients are very different. And this is why the distinct experiences of my patients and their feelings related to scoliosis treatment are reproduced verbatim below.

2 Patient Reports

The following Patient Reports are cited verbatim. Changes have only been made to passages describing treatment locations coming under criticism. Seen as a whole, these reports give a very good account as to what people afflicted with scoliosis feel. Adolescents describe how they experience brace treatment. Adults report how the intensive measures of in-patient rehabilitation have helped maintain their physical capacity.

It is also related that an operation may well be experienced without any complications if the patient has a positive attitude. However, two aspects become clear from these quite different descriptions:

The paths the individual patients pursue are very different, and getting-together with those similarly affected – for example, in a suitable support group or in in-patient rehabilitation – is deeply felt as sustaining and relieving.

What also becomes evident is the differences in treatment still existing today: Some braces seem to subject the patients to major discomfort, and that even without any good corrective effect, while other highly corrective provisions are described as pleasant.

Patient Report 6 is written extremely emotionally and portrays the emotional "roller-coaster ride" of some patients, which, while frequently experienced in a similar way, is seldom described so impressively. To begin with, I wondered whether I should take the liberty of publishing this report, since it might also be interpreted as revealing a lack of restraint. Ignoring for one moment the notion that my own work is perhaps underscored too much in this report, it may well also be of assistance to patients, particularly in view of the non-operative treatment of scoliosis patients that is still really backward abroad [i.e. not in Germany].

Due to the fact that this guidebook is also to be translated into other languages, I have quoted this report in the original. Two other Patient Reports are in the original language, the others translated from German with the usual adaptations being made.

Scoliosis Report No. 1

J. S. (16 years of age)

It was noticed with me shortly before Christmas in 2009. At that time I was still 14. One morning, when I was around at home in the rather tight T-shirt I wore at night, my father saw that something was up with me. My right shoulder-blade clearly protruded. I thought my father's wish to go to an orthopedist straightaway completely over the top. Nevertheless my mother quickly made an appointment at an orthopedist's. When he finally diagnosed that I had scoliosis, I was really knocked off my feet. He referred us to a very good address in his opinion. We were to call there and make an appointment ourselves. My mother was appalled that we had to wait four months for an appointment. This appointment unfortunately fell in the week of my practical work. My mother therefore canceled the appointment a little later and made a new one for two months later. My mother tried a great deal to get me an earlier appointment, but without any success. Then at last the time had come, and we set off early for the hospital. When we arrived there two hours later, I was first X-rayed. Then we were asked into the doctor's office. There we were able to see the X-ray, and I realized that I certainly had more than 20°. All the time I had secretly been hoping that I would not need a brace. I was well aware from my mother, who had since read up on the subject, that you needed a brace if you had over 20°. My concern was unfortunately confirmed when the doctor finally measured my X-ray and thus my curvature, and it turned out that I had 44° in my upper curvature and 34° in my lower one. But it was even worse when the doctor tried to encourage me in his indifferent manner by pointing out that I was still 6° away from an operation! He also told me directly that he couldn't do very much for me anyway, since I was already rather old - in the meantime 15 - for the brace treatment. I was also supposed to start doing another form of physical therapy, namely the one according to Schroth. Up until now I had only been prescribed normal physical therapy. Now to start with, a brace had to be constructed that I would then be wearing for 18 hours. To do this, we had to drive to the manufacturer to have a plaster cast made. After three weeks my brace was finally fitted. A lot had to be changed, and this was why it took quite some time before we were finished, which is, however, quite normal. In the end, the brace maker got his colleague to come and have a look at my brace. His first reaction was: "Does that shoulder blade ever stick out!" Finally, we could at last go home, and I was simply a nervous wreck. Back home, I immediately started with the process of getting used to wearing the brace. Here I had an additional challenge... namely, it was summer. To be exact, it was summer vacation, and it was hot. But for all intents and purposes, everything went well, and I had only "normal" pressure marks. However, it proved painful starting from a rib and spreading to my arm. Once when I moved my arm in the wrong direction while lying in bed, I had terrible pains in the rib that had already hurt when I was trying on the brace. Unfortunately, swelling soon developed there that was not visible in terms of color. So we drove back to the manufacturer. Here the brace was slightly modified, which, however, proved rather a challenge. They told us it could not be made much wider, since I had such a high degree value, and thus it was precisely the truss pad on my main curvature where the swelling had formed that was important. They also said that, in actual fact, even more pressure would have to be built up, since I had such a gigantic humped rib, after all. So we drove back home utterly devastated. Now I started having more and more difficulty sleeping. Often I took off the brace in the night without being aware of it. As these complaints simply did not cease and the swelling grew ever larger, we drove back to the hospital again. There the doctor examined me and said it was a hemorrhage. When we asked him what we could do about it, he said I leave the brace off for two weeks during the day and then try it again. So that's what I did, because I simply was at a loss to know what else to do. In the weeks without my brace, the swelling went down a bit. When I put the brace back on, it went right back to getting worse and bigger. We drove to the company a few times, only to be met with cluelessness there. We were also told that this complication is very rare – in only one of every 100 cases. Then it was time for the X-ray check. Here the doctor again examined my hemorrhage, and now he said it was peristonitis, which made me feel very unsettled. In response to the question as to what could be done about it, he simply said: "Nothing." The X-ray examination indicated that I only had a slight correction up above, which was why the pressure over my problem site had again increased. Unfortunately, this didn't improve matters. We now stopped going to the manufacturing company and doctor over and over. Meanwhile the pressure mark had already grown to the size of a hen's egg.

The pain made for very bad sleeping. On weekends, I always tore the brace from my body at 6 sharp and then mostly slept deeply until noon. This was very unusual for me, for I am, strictly speaking, an early-riser. At school, I now had problems with paying attention as well. Since the brace makers had said that a brace is never anything beautiful, I thought I just had to put up with it. In the meantime, my mother had been getting more information and discovered that there was another doctor with a good reputation. She tried to persuade me to go there, though I didn't want to at first. Even my father thought it was a good idea, especially because he had noticed that my humped rib was visibly more and more pronounced. When my mother had at last persuaded me, we got an appointment in a matter of two weeks. And so we went to the new doctor's office (though I had mixed feelings about it). At first, this doctor was very surprised by my reserved greeting. You could also say that I was somewhat intimidated by the host of nice men who had been treating me up till then. This doctor was completely different from the previous one. He actually talked with me and had a good, close look at my brace. It turned out that it was too small, which, in turn, made it clear to me why I had been feeling nauseous and hardly able to eat anything. He also said that this brace was certainly not the worst he'd ever seen, but not the best either. He suggested we have a new brace made immediately - at the company right there. True, I did hesitate, but then readily agreed, as my parents were totally convinced. Here, too, I was also told that there wasn't much more they could do for me, and the doctor said it was up to me whether I wanted a brace at all. Thus, it was entirely my own decision. It was said that they would be able to accomplish something in terms of appearance, and that was the precise reason why I said yes. For the very first time since the start of my treatment, I did not feel like I was seriously ill. I was X-rayed and had achieved a slight improvement in my degree values through the old brace. So I went right over to the new company. Here, the treatment was completely different from the old one as well. I was constantly being asked whether it was all right with me if some changes had to be made, with me always answering in the affirmative, totally bewildered. They hurried it up a good deal, and so my new brace was ready for fitting after just two weeks. I was fitted with the trial brace, and I went directly to the doctor with it on, for I'd been told he always wanted to see the trial brace worn. It surprised me very much that it fit me so well the first time around, which had not been the case with any of my braces up till then. The doctor himself marked where something had to be altered. A brace maker from the company was also in attendance. Then we went to the company, and it was adjusted. Here, everyone was again very polite and treated me much more courteously than had been the case with the older company. I also had my X-ray check behind me by now and was feeling much better. It turned out that I now had a much better correction on top, and quite a bit had also happened in terms of appearance. Naturally, I had pressure marks, but they were bearable. Although my peristonitis had since receded, it had left hardening (sclerosis) behind. Part of it had already been transformed into bone. This will probably never go away, which, however, does not disturb me. I was truly astonished, for – despite the fact that I had been wearing my new brace almost right from the outset for 23 hours – the inflammation has gone down. It was really high time for a change, since the constant inflammation had very much weakened my immune system and caused me to have ongoing colds. My psyche also suffered very much. My mother and my friends say that, since having my new brace, I again have more vitality, more zest for life, which is obvious to me, too, of course. What has really helped me is that I've since told my class that I have to wear a brace and can therefore be much more open now. Right at the start, I only told my good friends. Meanwhile, my entire circle of acquaintances knows about it, and they've all reacted really well. More than anything, my report goes to show that you should never delay in getting several opinions if you entertain any doubts as to whether the treatment is the right one. I am very satisfied with my decision and also with my appearance. Nobody notices my scoliosis, and I can even, for example, go to the swimming pool without any fear. An operation would never come into question for me. In the meantime, I have also been to a health resort, where I made friends with some other girls. I am quite good at physical therapy exercises now, too. I think that the brace is most important for me, although my two hours of physical therapy are also very helpful. Here I do the exercises with another girl I've become friends with and who also wears a brace. We understand each other well and are happy to be able to talk about our special problems for once. I think I can be really satisfied, and I'm grateful that in the severe initial period of my scoliosis treatment, my animals, my friends, and my family helped me so much. I have accepted my scoliosis and know that I can live with it, which is why I'm doing so much better.

Scoliosis Report No. 2
H. A. (16 years of age)

The diagnosis of a brace came as a real bombshell to me. It was a shock that I couldn't quite grasp. Two years earlier, I had completed a special muscle-building training program for my back due to my crooked spinal column. Yet now it was determined that it had been applied at the wrong point, and only a brace could save me from further deterioration and thus perhaps from spinal fusion as well. While I was not yet aware at that moment how this would affect my life in the future, endless questions nevertheless shot through my head: Can I still live a normal life with my brace? To what extent will the brace affect me in everyday life and in school? And perhaps the most important question for me at the time: Can I still keep playing the competitive sport I love so much? After his diagnosis, my orthopedist referred me to a specialist, who made my worst foreboding come true: He made it unmistakably clear to me that competitive sports and braces are not compatible, and I would therefore have to quit. However, I could not and did not want to accept this – out of love for my sport, for one thing, and, for another, since all doctors up till now had said that my sport was good for my back. For this reason I wanted to hear a second opinion, and through my neighbor's wife, who also wears a brace, I came to a second specialist. He made a very nice impression and explained to me that I would not have to give up my sport at all. However, he did recommend – in addition to the brace – that I get involved in special back therapy: physical therapy according to Schroth. What is more, I was to go to a health resort to learn the physical therapy properly in order to be able to continue it at home on my own. He then fitted me with a brace with the aid of a plaster cast. At this point in time, I was not aware that this was an obsolete method and would lead to considerable problems down the line. After a period of three to four weeks of getting used to it, I was to wear the brace 16 hours a day. But even the first attempts at getting accustomed to it made me lose all hope of ever feeling happy with a brace. I couldn't bear it for more than one hour on any given day and then had such severe pain that I was unable to do anything at all. Even at night it was not any better, as I would wake up from to the pain every half hour and then could not sleep any more, even if I took off the brace at some point. Still I tried it again and again, hoping that it would perhaps work out somehow. Yet this merely led to sleep deprivation, causing my academic and athletic performance to suffer considerably. I was unable to properly concentrate any longer and was tired all the time. For this reason, we arranged a new appointment with the doctor and described my situation to him. But he only told me that I would ultimately get used to it. After six months, however, it was still no better. By chance I happened to talk with my math teacher about my situation and my problems with the brace. He told me that his two daughters likewise wore braces but had no problems whatsoever with them. He gave me the address of their doctor, a Dr. Weiss, whom we made an appointment with as quickly as possible. In our first talks, Dr. Weiss immediately made a very nice, personable, and above all insightful impression and determined that my brace had been fitted much too small. This presumably had to do with the obsolete method. For this reason, he fitted me with a new brace with the aid of scanners and various further measurements. My newly kindled hope was directly rewarded the first time I wore the brace: I did not have any pain any more for the very first time. After some "fine tuning," Dr. Weiss was satisfied, and so was I. The prescribed period of wear of 16–20 hours suddenly no longer posed a problem, and I could again sleep through the night without pain. My academic performance stabilized, and I can look forward to finishing high school without a worry. Even my athletic performance was no longer adversely affected – in fact, practically the opposite is true: This year, despite the brace, I was able to qualify for the European championships for the first time ever, which is the biggest success of my whole career so far. In conclusion, I can only recommend the following to anyone who has to wear a brace: Never accept a brace that causes pain. A brace is not intended to be a great impairment, except in a certain respect naturally looking slightly bulky and affecting some movements a little. You only have to purchase some new clothes for the brace to fit underneath. You get used to the rest really fast, and for the success you accomplish, these are marginal sacrifices of no real significance.

Scoliosis Report No. 3

C. S. (15 years of age)

I was in 6th grade when my scoliosis was diagnosed. At that time, I was 12 years old and had a curvature of 43°. I thought it wasn't anything bad and that it would go away on its own. Of course, it was nothing like that at all. I was told I'd get a brace. At first, I had no idea what this was. When I looked up orthopedic brace on the Internet, I was initially shocked. So this was what I was supposed to wear?

About two weeks later, I was at the orthopedist's, who handed me my first brace about a week later. It was quite manageable to wear it in winter, although I got back sores. What really drove me crazy, however, were the brackets reaching to the collarbone. All T-shirts therefore had to be high-necked. What's more, I noticed after a few weeks that my leg kept falling asleep after sitting in the brace for a long time, causing an unpleasant pulling sensation right up the back. After about 18 months and numerous adaptations and alterations, it did not fit at all anymore.

I had my second brace made at another doctor's. He was reputedly better. I was straightaway encased in plaster there (a god-awful feeling). After one week, the second brace was then ready to use. It was only about half as big as the previous one and was reminiscent of a very large, white plastic belt. But this brace had drawbacks as well. It was made of very thick plastic and also fully plastered with thick and hard truss pads that led to pressure marks. I was not satisfied with this brace either, especially because it did not really improve the curvature. When this brace no longer fit, I got a third one (again from a different doctor). Once again, it turned out quite differently. It was larger, made of thinner plastic, and was generally more pleasant to wear than the previous ones. I have now had this brace for around two years. This last one has helped the most and has definitely improved the curvature more than the others.

Fortunately, none of the three braces could be seen through my clothing, and I was always able to wear what I wanted. And so it ended up that many in my class who knew have forgotten about the brace and today are quite surprised when I tell them that I am still wearing it. I always used to wear each brace at school and also at night, but never 23 hours a day. I managed to wear it at the most 18 to 20 hours a day. This is due to the fact that it proved annoying both when studying as well as at meals, as it quickly became to restrictive for me. Although the wearing period was shorter than prescribed, my back still improved, since I regularly went to physical therapy. What's more, I attended a two-hour course that taught me how to correct my posture in everyday life whenever I'm not wearing the brace. Now I only have to wear it for 16 hours. This means I only have to wear it at school and at night. Wearing a brace is anything but fun, yet – with the right attitude and good friends – you can manage to make it through this time passably. Getting involved in a lot of sports is very important (after all, here you can take off the brace, for "Sport = support"). My recommendation: Simply try to do everything that you used to do without the brace, but a little bit modified.

Scoliosis Report No. 4
K. Y. (17 years of age, Moscow)

My name is Katharina; I am 17 years old and come from Russia. I would like to start my story from the very moment I was diagnosed with "scoliosis." It all began during ballet lessons in January 2006, when I was 13 years of age. My teacher noticed that the left part of my back was slightly higher than the right and recommended that I see an orthopedist. My parents soon found a doctor in Moscow to help me. The doctor was not unfriendly, but his words left me fearful and crying. My scoliosis came to 22°. He said that nowadays there were two ways of treating it: the conservative treatment or an operation should the curvature continue to increase. I did not want either – I just wanted to get away again quickly and forget everything. The doctor was of the opinion that it was not so bad with me and gave me hope that the treatment would not last long.

My parents managed to calm me down, explaining to me that everyone has difficulties in life sometime or other and that it's not possible to avoid it. There is probably no such thing as complete good health, and there are cases that simply cannot be cured. At any rate, they went on to say, I had a chance of improving my curvature and should take advantage of it.

I was sent to a health resort in Moscow, where there were children and adolescents with the widely varying degrees of curvature. The doctors at this health resort worked out individual exercise programs. I was forced to get involved in gymnastics for one hour a day over a period of one month, and then I had massages and electrostimulation, then gymnastics again. This was how the days passed, but in between I also had time to eat and recuperate, as well as for the school and for friends. At the health resort, a plaster bed was prepared for me that I had to sleep in. To tell the truth, it was heavy and ultimately unsuitable. I was made a KPO-14 brace as well, which was of no help. I spent a month at the health resort. Back home, we immediately consulted the doctor, and I expected to hear words to like: "Everything is back to normal. You're healthy again." Instead of which, except for muscular growth, nothing had obviously changed.

It was then that my parents decided to look for other potential treatment. My father started to research scoliosis more intensively, reading books on the subject as well as searching for information on the Internet, including in forums. It was thanks to his efforts that I heard of the Chêneau brace and of a specialist in Germany. Without my father, it's a sure thing that I never would have found out about this.

We therefore decided to go to Germany to a consultation with this specialist and also to have a brace made there. As it turned out, I already had 42° at the bottom and 33° at the top. The specialist was sure that he could help us. This gave me great hope. He sent us to the orthopedics workshop where we were able to select the Chêneau light brace. To tell the truth, I was shocked that I had to wear it for more than 20 hours, and I was also worried as to what my friends would have to say about it. I know today that it was not a matter of their opinion, but of my life. My parents helped me again to take the right step. They explained to me that I can be proud of the brace and don't need to be ashamed of it. If anyone asks what it is, I can also simply and boldly reply that it is a brace to get well again. This is how I lived for three years. Most of the people did not even notice the brace at all. I wore it at least 20 hours every day, and it was not difficult at all. I only took it off for physical education and when showering. In winter it was very easy to put up with, especially under the turtlenecks; in summer it was a little hot, which is why I sometimes did not put it on during the day. I traveled to Germany to the specialist for a check-up twice a year, and the results pleased me more and more, because the degree values became increasingly lower. After the first month of brace treatment, the curvature was only 25° at the top and 23° at the bottom; after one year in the next brace, 19° top and 0 bottom. After treatment ended, I now have – without the brace – 35° top and 31° bottom; however, I have also avoided the operation.

Scoliosis Report No. 5
S. H. (19 years of age)

It was in 2007 when I went to my family doctor one day at noon to go through the usual general youth physical exam. I had already noticed that my back was not quite straight; however, I had not given it any serious thought at this time. My family doctor also noticed my slightly crooked back and referred me to an orthopedist just to be sure I did not have any serious back problems. I went to the orthopedist with mixed feelings, who determined scoliosis at 20°. Due to the fact that I'd never heard anything of scoliosis up till now, the initial shock was very great! What precisely was wrong with my back? How bad was it? My orthopedist prescribed me physical therapy once a week.

After some time, I went to see my orthopedist again to have him determine what effect the physical therapy had had on my spine. Completely confident, I entered the doctor's office to hear my scoliosis had worsened by 10°. A course of treatment or a brace would be necessary to counter any curvature progression. A doctor specializing in scoliosis was recommended to me. I left the orthopedist crying my eyes out. I thought my whole life was destroyed and I had a horrible disease. Full of fear and anxiety, I set out to see this doctor. Although he prescribed me a course of treatment AND a brace, after the talk with him I felt much better! He had such an amazing way of advising me, calming my fears, giving me courage, and showing me that, on the one hand, scoliosis is not a severe illness, and, on the other, that many more people suffer from such degrees of curvature than you think. With his empathetic way, he gained my trust. I felt immediately in good hands with him and knew that he understood my worries and anxieties.

I got my brace that same year. It was a so-called Chêneau light brace. The brace makers were very kind and understanding as well. They quickly convinced me that I should regard the brace as my helper and not as a monster, and so I rapidly became friends with my new daily companion, wearing it every day for 20 hours without any problems. I only felt pain on the first day and never again after that. I got used to my brace very fast, and I didn't find the nights at all bad either. For me, it was – to be quite honest – the reverse: It was much for me to get used to going to bed again without plastic. There were no problems with the people around me. Right away, I showed the brace to others quite openly, and from then on it was part of me, like eyeglasses are for other people. The worst aspect of my brace was the heat. Sometimes, when the upper part of my body was once again soaking wet from sweat, I would have just as soon ripped off the brace and thrown it away. But I always managed to remain persistent and rational, constantly reminding myself that I was doing this for me and that I didn't want to regret it later that I'd been inconsistent. This optimistic attitude was really important in successfully achieving my good health. It was thanks to the support from my family that I was able to develop such optimism!

In the summer of the same year (2008), I went to attend a five-week course of treatment. The Schroth gymnastics used there, the motivating therapists, and the all of the other patients did me and my back the world of good! I got to know a girl at the clinic who is still a very good friend of mine now, three years later, and who can simply understand me with my scoliosis better than anyone. I also met some other girls with braces that were really big and very heavy. While it is true that it was said that these braces were slightly more effective than the Chêneau light brace, I did observe, however, that many of these orthoses mostly lay around in the room, since they caused terrible back pain. For this reason, I was pleased that I possessed a brace with a light-weight design, since I was able to wear it 20 hours a day – as prescribed – and therefore attained greater efficiency.

After the health treatment, I did my exercises at home every day, and once a week I was helped by a therapist. During a check-up, my doctor established that both the brace as well as the treatment at the health resort had contributed towards considerably improving my scoliosis. After one more examination, it was apparent that I was fully grown and could therefore slowly get used to not wearing my brace.

Now I have survived everything and am really proud of my mastering this time so amazingly! The handicap strengthened me a great deal mentally and made me more confident!

Finally, I would like to express my thanks to my doctor, the brace makers at the company, my family, and naturally my brace (which, incidentally, I have hung up in my room as a souvenir).

And I should like to pass on my doctor's tip to every patient: If you don't let your scoliosis drive you crazy, but enjoy life instead, everything is half as bad!

Scoliosis Report No. 6
S. B. (15 years old, New Zealand)

I still remember it ever so clearly, imprinted in my memory. December 2008. When I saw Dr Hans Rudolf Weiss for the very first time. This is a day that cannot easily be forgotten, a day with much significance. A day which changed my life.

I came to Dr. Weiss as a late developing 12 year old girl, with a scoliosis of approximately 35 degrees that was rapidly increasing. He told me not to worry, because a spinal brace worn 23/d would be able to put a halt to the progression of the curvature, and correct it to an extent. Hearing this I was drowned in an ocean of emotions – largely happiness, uncertainty and fear. Would this alternative solution really work? Does this man know what he's doing? Will my life be different wearing this brace for the next couple of years, 23/d? The answer to all of my initial questions is yes. This wave of sensations triggered the response of tears. Tears which were empty and had no meaning. I can quote Dr. Weiss, who had quite obviously observed this reaction many times before as he said – "mark my words child, once you have matured, those tears will be nothing but the tears of joy." The man was right. Two and a half years later I am writing this. And yes. Yes I did experience those tears of joy. But how did I end up in this rewarding position?

The moment I stepped out of the patients room, I realized that it was me, and me alone on a journey along an unknown road. I knew where the start was, and where the final destination would hopefully be. I did not know how long it would take, or how it would impact on my life. There was much help and support by my side from friends, family and professionals, however, in the end it comes down to you and the decisions you make. I am not going to lie – there were several bumps along this road, and some aspects of it were more pleasurable than others. I walked down this road and took it step by step. From the start I was aware of the different places my journey could end depending on how I coped with my scoliosis. Obviously, pure out of human nature, I strived for the best possible final destination. The best possible result. In order to achieve this desired outcome, I had to do everything in my ability, as I knew it would not come naturally.

This is a story about my journey of living with scoliosis. My name is Sanne, and I am an average New Zealand girl who likes the outdoors, surfing, hanging out with friends, and playing tennis. Life was good. And remained good, much to my surprise. When I was 12, I had a 15 degree curve which progressed to a double curve of 25 degrees at the bottom and 20 degrees at the top, in a period of just 6 months. I then started an intense exercise scheme for the next 3 months, 4 times per week. By now I was 12 and three quarters and my curvature had increased to 30 degrees at the bottom and 35 degrees at the top. The intense exercise programme had obviously not worked, and I was running out of options apart from the operation. My mother then went online and found the help I needed in Germany from Dr. Weiss. The specialists in New Zealand advised us against going there as they do not so much believe in bracing and exercising methods to correct scoliosis. Thanks to my mothers stubbornness, she insisted we buy plane tickets to Germany that very same day. I went to Germany at the age of 12 and 10 months over the Christmas period. We soon saw Dr. Weiss which takes me back to my first encounter with him, when he told me about wearing the Chêneau-lite brace until I had fully matured. At the time I believed that my world had turned upside down and collapsed. But just like most things – it wasn't nearly as bad as it seemed. After a month, I left back for New Zealand with a well fitting brace, a exercise routine and a whole new positive attitude towards correcting my scoliosis.

Once I got back it took me a couple of weeks to get used to living in this brace. I still went to the beach and did what I would normally do over the summer.

Then came my first day at high school which was nerve racking enough by itself, but with a brace my nervousness doubled. And once again – it was not as bad as I had imagined. My school uniform fitted perfectly with my brace, and it wasn't noticeable for others to see that I was wearing a brace. To be completely honest – I was extremely self-conscious of my brace as it made me "different" to the rest. I heard many stories about teenagers who showed off their back braces in and out of school. I absolutely respected those people, and wished that I had the guts to do the same.

Instead I covered it all up. In fact, I was so conscious about my brace I only told 3 of my close friends who kept it secret. The Physical Education teacher was the only other person at school who knew. No one else ever noticed me wearing a back brace, over a period of one and a half years. I still wonder how people could not have noticed – perhaps because no one expects it as they have never heard of a back brace before, or perhaps they seemed more absorbed in their own world, or maybe I just made a bigger deal of it than it really was inside my head? Most teenagers have an obsession with appearance, but that was not so much my reason for covering up my brace. My biggest fear was that people would find out and treat me differently – as though I had a handicap. Now from experience I know that his would not have happened, yet I do believe that it is best if one tells the world about their scoliosis only if they are comfortable with the concept – remember, nobody is perfect and everyone has their differences. Of course I had to make several adaptations to my normal life by wearing this brace, but they were minimal. Like a drop of water in a lake. The drop of water being the few short-term changes, and the lake being a whole lifetime. So after about half a year of wearing my brace full time I went back to Germany to get my brace adjusted, and then I went back yet again, a year after that at the age of 14 and a half. This is when I gradually started wearing my brace less over the winter period and in 6 months, by the time it was summer (end of 2010) I was down to wearing my brace only at night. I saw Dr. Weiss for what may have been the last time ever in July 2011. He said I no longer had to wear my brace – not even at night as I had matured. My spine is back to 15 degrees at the bottom and 20 degrees at the top.

What a beautiful closure. Doctor Weiss is a man who speaks the truth. This is the moment the tears of joy were provoked. For me it was a very hard goodbye. I did not only say goodbye to Dr. Weiss and the brace maker Mr. Werkmann, but also to my brace – the thing that significantly improved my life. I still don't know why it was so hard letting go of my brace – as though I was leaving behind part of myself. Literally. Wearing this brace is the best decision I have ever made and it worked out better than expected. Now I have a relatively straight spine without any pain – and I owe it all to Dr. Weiss. Someone who changes many lives, and does it from his heart, not for the money. So I guess my journey ends here, in a small German village. More than 18,000 kilometers from home. My final destination has been reached.

Lots of love from "Down Under" Sanne

Scoliosis Report No. 7
(B. B., 15 years old)

It all started on a sunny spring day in April 2003, a spring of change and uncertainty...

Due to the back pain that I had every evening, I went to my family doctor to have myself examined. Deep down inside me, I was very sure that it would not be anything bad and that it perhaps involved too much strain on my back. The doctor had me do the forward bend test and quite clearly saw that I had scoliosis. At first, I didn't know at all what it is or what it looks like. My family doctor made an urgent appointment with an orthopedist. I was still hoping that it would not be scoliosis, although I still did not know precisely what that is. I did the forward bend test again, and, in order to be quite sure, X-rays were also taken. But the diagnosis was the same: scoliosis. I could see on the X-ray images what scoliosis looks like, but nobody explained anything in any detail to me. Physical therapy was prescribed for me. I could not come to terms with the diagnosis and called on a second orthopedist, who had treated me once before. The diagnosis was the same. This is when I heard for the first time what scoliosis actually is.

My family doctor had already pointed out to me at the first exam that I might have to wear a brace. I now hoped that it would not turn out that I only got lucky once on this day. Not a chance! I was prescribed a brace and physical therapy according to Katharina Schroth. Even today, it is still hard for me to explain what was going on inside me at this moment...

I was released from physical education for my remaining time at school. For some other scoliosis patients, sports means a great deal, but not for me. Yet occasionally I did miss really getting wild with my friends and not always having to be different. Despite my great reluctance, I went to physical therapy twice a week. At the beginning, this was nothing but a waste of time for me. I did not understand at all what everyone expected of me – as far as I was concerned, my back was straight. As the summer slowly came to an end, I realized they were right. When I looked at myself in the mirror, I immediately saw that my back was not as straight as I had always thought. It was certainly no simple task for my physiotherapists to get me to have this sense of my body.

When fall began, which meant that my physiotherapy came to an end as well, thoughts of my scoliosis simply vanished. It was only rarely that I thought of it. Until the day when the appointment for fitting my brace was made. I drove with my mother to this appointment – long awaited on her part and absolutely detested on mine. I was also afraid, as I didn't know what I was getting into or what was going to happen to me. A medical team welcomed me and discussed the procedure with me. I had to put on a white shirt and was then encased in plaster. When the plaster got increasingly hotter and harder, I almost started panicking. After three hours, my mother drove me back home.

Winter eventually came, and Christmas was around the corner. I was called by the medical supply store and told that my brace was ready to be picked up. I was curious. What would it look like? But when I saw this thing for the first time, I was close to tears. At that moment I was simply speechless. A few details were altered, and then I was able to go back home. Hardly had I arrived home when the thing landed in the nearest corner. I fought wearing it tooth and nail. I hated it – I thought of it as a monster! It pinched all over. I could hardly move - I didn't want to be so restricted! I wanted to be just like other people! It took a long time for me to come to terms with the fact that I'm not like everybody else! That I can't move as freely as I want. At the start, I never wore the brace. But sometime or other the day arrived when I told myself that I was doing this for myself and my life, and for nobody else. All the same, it was difficult to put up with the brace to begin with; it was painful, and I had to learn how to adapt my movements to accomplish certain everyday things. Now more than a year has gone by. I've been grappling with scoliosis a great deal, reading reports and books and trying to get in touch with others. It has often been hard, and there will certainly be more difficult times for me ahead. But all of this has very much shaped my life. I often recall the day my scoliosis was diagnosed and the day when I myself realized that a whole lot would change.

Finally, I would like to write a few words to all those who are afflicted: For some it is easier to deal with scoliosis, for others more difficult. I believe I belong to the second category. But I would like to tell everyone: Don't give up living! Even if it's hard to get up again when you've landed flat on your back. I know how hard it is to put up with clever sayings like this. I, too, have often wished that all those who used to poke fun at me would be stuck in this brace just for one day – to experience with their own body how hard it is to suddenly be unable to move freely. It is by no means a simple thing to keep finding the strength to tell yourself: You are doing this for yourself and for nobody else.

I also think some will ask themselves the same question I did: Why me, of all people? I feel sure that one day the time will come when all our sacrifice and limitations will have been worthwhile, and also that we will be able to freely move again. All of us will always remain affected by scoliosis, and for the rest of our lives we will certainly never forget what we've experienced with it! Yet I think that even this period will sometime belong to the past. There are so many afflicted by scoliosis in this world, and this one fate links us all.

Here's wishing you all the very best! B. B.

Scoliosis Report No. 8

S. T. (15 years of age)

"My bracey and me"

I was 11when my mother noticed my crooked spine, since she herself has scoliosis. In her case, it was first discovered when she was 15, and she had gymnastic exercises prescribed. She has been doing her exercises up to the present day, or else she has pain. When I was at the orthopedist's for the first time, he said it might straighten out again in the course of my growing. In those days, I almost never thought about it. On my next visit, he spoke of an operation. That was why we changed to another orthopedist to hear his opinion. That was the right thing to do, as it turned out. There was no more talk of an operation. I was again under observation, and I kept on going to my gymnastics exercises every week. By this time I was 13 and attending 8th grade in secondary school. In early 2003, I was once again in the orthopedist's waiting room without a clue as to what would happen. When she then measured the degree value of my curvature on the X-ray and had a look at my back, she said I would be getting a brace. I had 21°, and I was almost fully grown. That was the biggest shock of my life; I simply could not believe it, and didn't want to either!

To be honest, I was terrified. But now nothing could be done about it. If I was still against it after giving it some thought, I was to go to a health resort. And did I ever give it some thought! I didn't think of anything else. I hardly spoke at all on that day, but only cried. I thought it was the end of my life of freedom. What on earth can I even do in a brace? 23 hours, every day – it all seemed like just a nightmare. Gradually, everyone found out about it - my family and my friends. Everyone tried to comfort me: I would get through it and they would always be there for me. I did not have the feeling that I would make it, but I had to!

It got closer to the time. After a plaster cast, my brace was made. It was to be fitted at the hospital on 4/14/2003. That was my mother's 34th birthday and my grandmother's birthday as well. The night before, everyone had called or texted me. I was petrified, but at the same time somehow also curious about my brace and the other girl in my room. Was she nice? Just a few hours of freedom left! When we had arrived, I had first gone from doctor to doctor filling out forms. I found the hospital quite OK. My room was also nice with a view of the woods. I said goodbye to my mother, but fortunately my companion in suffering was already there. Her name was Katja, and she was 15 years old. Katja was really very nice, and we got along super together. We not only shared the room, but also our trials and tribulations. I now had my brace, and to begin with I couldn't walk or sit properly. Everything was so weird – it was also very painful. Now I was in a cage. We were given balls to sit on. The first night I could not lie down at all; everything hurt, and I slept again without the brace. The week passed by quite quickly; although I didn't always do so well, I slowly got used to the idea of having to wear it all the time. By the way, I had started to call my brace "bracey," which was a good sign, I think.

Back home, everyone was naturally curious about my bracey, and duly horrified when they saw it. But they all stuck with me, and helped me wherever they could. Slowly but surely the pain subsided, but so did my self-confidence. Practically all my clothing no longer fit me. I could only wear other things. I always had the feeling that others could see it, which was precisely what I didn't want at all. In my class, everyone looked at me when I had to go up front to the board. But they were only inquisitive and would never have laughed at me or teased me. Rather, they admired how well I handled all of this. But what they didn't know was what was going on inside of me. At school, I withdrew a bit; I even swore to myself that I wouldn't have any friends during this time, because I could not imagine anyone understanding it. But if you love somebody, then you love this person the way he or she is. In the end, I actually did have a friend, which I'm sure was a big help to me. Naturally, I would have preferred to throw in the towel a thousand times over, but I knew that I had to get through it, and also that I could.

The worst part was the summer, because it was so hot and the others were running around in bikinis. Every time we went back to the doctor, I expected her to say that at last my spine was straight again and that I was done with my bracey. But things dragged on, and winter came. At least everyone was wearing thick clothing anyway.

Then I was told the date when I would start to gradually wean myself off of bracey: on 2/9/2004. I'm already counting the days until it's finally time. Because my biggest wish is to celebrate my 15th birthday without bracey. But I would never have dreamed that I would be rid of it by then.

I must say that I am rather proud of myself for surviving this difficult time. For it was not only hard for myself, but also for my parents and the rest of my family, I'm sure. I would like to thank my family and friends for always being there for me, for sticking with me and supporting me. I would never have made it without them. This was also how I discovered what true friends are, namely those who are always there for you and also stick with you in had times. A whole new life will soon be starting for me. Before, I did not know how to appreciate some things at all. Sleeping on my back or stomach again, not on hard plastic, and especially putting on clothes my own size again. I only saw my bracey as evil and not that it was helping me. However, I do know this now, which is why I am thankful for it. I shall never forget it and will certainly think of it often and be grateful all over again.

Scoliosis Report No. 9

(U. M., 58 years of age)

35 years ago, I was diagnosed with onsetting scoliosis that has been treated conservatively ever since that time. Today, the condition has unfortunately progressed so far that the right-convex lumbar scoliosis has attained a curvature of 50° acc. to Cobb, and I suffer from chronic pains; what is more, kyphosis ("humpback") has developed in the last two years as well. The last course of treatment, from 02/01 to 02/22/2006, did not result in any improvement. The wish I expressed when applying for the course of treatment that I would be admitted to a special clinic would have made more sense, in my opinion, because special exercises for scoliosis patients are offered there. This was confirmed when a therapist said, "We rarely see patients with such pronounced curvature."

On the recommendation of an acquaintance, I consulted Dr. med. Weiss, who, after an in-depth examination, prescribed the "physiologic-brace," paid for by my health insurance.

Today I can report that after 15 hours of consistent use each day over a period of six months, the pain has been alleviated. As recommended, I set aside the brace for about a month, hoping the effects on pain relief and mobility that had been attained would last. However, the pains and instability resumed after about two months, so now I'm constantly wearing the brace again. I am grateful, however, that this resource exists, since it has restored my quality of life to an extent.

I can go on two-hour hikes again and even take part in evening social events, which was no longer possible without the brace. Nevertheless, I also have to continue shoring up this regained mobility by doing sports activities such as swimming and daily Schroth therapy with at least one period of rest a day.

It is my hope that, thanks to this report on my experience, more patients with the same condition as mine will be reimbursed for the cost of a "physiologic-brace" by their health insurance.

Scoliosis Report No. 10

K. A. (16 years of age)

I was diagnosed with scoliosis when I was 12 years old. At that time, it was only 12 degrees in the main curvature. I was only prescribed physical therapy up until I was 13. During this time, my scoliosis worsened by 20 degrees. I was then provided with a brace. I wore it 23 hours a day on a regular basis. Nevertheless, my spinal column worsened by 15 degrees. From then on, I only wore my brace very rarely and no pursued physical therapy as intensively as at the beginning. I simply lost all interest in working on my spinal column, since none of my efforts had been worthwhile.

When I was 15, walking or standing for longer periods was painful for me, so I finally asked my doctor where and how I could be operated on. Shortly after that, I checked in to the hospital. The main curvature measured at 60 degrees. I was then admitted as an inpatient in December 1997.

Before the operation, I was taught how to stand and lie down properly after the operation. Otherwise, only the usual preparations and examinations were carried out.

December 16th was the big day. I ended up not being very anxious, as the doctors had explained to me in great detail what would be happening during and after the operation. I had also heard from my orthopedist that the risk of paraplegia had been almost 0% at this hospital for 30 years.

Nine vertebrae were fused, i.e. two screws were inserted into each vertebra, with the intervertebral disks replaced by titanium cages filled with pelvic bone. Finally, a rod is passed through the screws. This rod straightens the spinal column and prevents the vertebrae from slipping back into the old position.

When I returned to my ward after 5 days in intensive care, I had to get up and walk twice a day with the physical therapists. At first, I was only able to sit and walk for 5 minutes. I did notice, however, it kept getting better from day to day. (After my operation, I did not have a brace or even a cast.) When I was discharged 4 weeks later, I went right back to school (only for a few hours at a time to begin with) to get myself used to everyday life as fast as possible. Now, 10 months later, I feel as if I had never been operated on. I am mobile, go regularly to school, go out, and exercise.

Sometimes if I have to sit for longer than 8 hours, I do have slight pain, but that is normal in the first year after the operation.

I can only advise anyone who has decided or is still thinking about it to go to the hospital for outpatient consultation as soon as possible. This is because each scoliosis case is unique and is operated on differently as well. But each person has to know whether he or she can handle the pain after the operation. It is not a simple procedure, such as a tonsillectomy, and so you should be very well informed concerning the doctors, hospitals, and surgery options beforehand.

As someone afflicted with scoliosis, you are very much dependent on good physical therapists, brace makers, and physicians.

I am completely satisfied, and can say: "I'd prefer being operated on ten more times to wearing a brace again. It was totally unnecessary." I really have to tell you what a truly amazing feeling it was to be able to put on close-fitting T-shirts this summer without thinking about how best to hide my "package."

So through my operation I have regained some self-confidence and my "quality of life."

Scoliosis Report No. 11
(L. M., 15 years of age)

It was precisely five years ago when I started having this problem. I was 10 at the time, and at first I didn't think much of anything was wrong. But I later saw in the mirror that I didn't stand up straight, and many other adults and children noticed it as well. So an orthopedist was recommended to us. The orthopedist explained to me that I had scoliosis. He advised me to go to a medical practice for physical therapy and massage twice a week. Meanwhile, we heard about a clinic in Aachen. The doctor there did not exactly encourage me and determined that I absolutely had to have a brace. This made me very sad and stunned at the same time. We found an orthopedist, who said that, while he did not yet have experience treating this problem in children, he wanted to try, and in a short time he had a brace made for me. I wore this brace for six months.

My mother then found a rehab clinic on the Internet. We called there straightaway and applied for a course of treatment that was to last four weeks. This treatment helped me an awful lot, since we did a great many different Schroth exercises several times a day. Initially, it was hard for me to understand how to do the exercises and especially the special breathing technique, but I mastered it in next to no time. At the clinic, I was given a new brace because the old one from the orthopedist pinched at the wrong points. Naturally, my face gave away how disappointed I was. My family and I very much regretted having a brace made by someone who was not experienced in treating scoliosis in children. Still, I did not want to give up, and since I had made such great strides by the end of the treatment thanks to the exercises, I planned to repeat it the following year. I switched to another practice and am still going to see a therapist who does the same exercises with me that I learned during the course of treatment. Fortunately, this has helped as well and, though often strenuous, has been a great deal of fun.

At the same time, we go to the orthopedist at the rehab clinic for a check-up every three months.

Two years passed by, and I didn't have one single complaint about the brace. When we went back after a few months for the regular brace check-up, we were told that my supervising doctor was no longer working at the clinic. At first we were upset, especially because we had not been informed either in writing or by phone. But since we didn't know if and where my orthopedist was working at first, there was nothing else we could do but have a new brace made at the clinic, since the old one was too small. At every brace checkup, I was always told that my scoliosis had not deteriorated, but had remained the same or even improved. After that, I was more hopeful than ever and wore the brace many hours a day.

I wore the new brace for one and a half years. It was only then that we received a letter with the address of my former doctor. We went there just a few weeks later, and it was determined using an X-ray that I had deteriorated by 20° within one and a half years. Tears welled up, and I had an indescribably terrible feeling, for a 75° curvature was anything but a joke. The doctor was of the opinion that the brace made at the clinic was not correct, and a new one for me at his practice. I also went to see two therapists, who went through various everyday activities with me and showed me things like how to sit at school. This has helped me enormously. I can stand the new brace a lot better, and it was not at all hard for me to wear it at school for a year. All in all, I determined to keep the brace on not less than twenty hours and do at least half an hour of Schroth exercises at home on my wall bars every day.

I hope that I will have much more success with the new brace and wish that everyone with the same problem as I have will not give up getting their scoliosis under control as fast as possible!

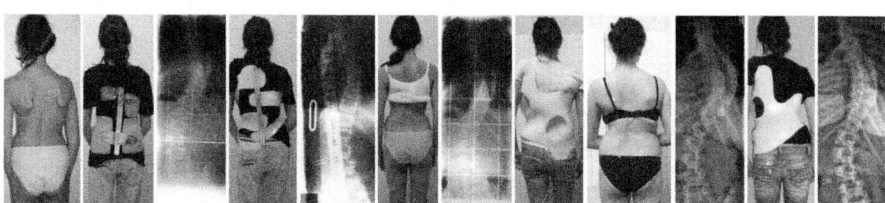

Scoliosis Report No. 12

Here is my story (KF, 17 years)

When I was nine, my mother noticed that my spine was not straight, although I was actively participating in ballet, tennis, and swimming. My mother took me to my pediatrician's office, and after he checked, he said that nothing was wrong. A year later, my mother took me back to the doctor's office and insisted to order an X-ray. The X-ray showed a significant spinal curvature. I started taking physical therapy, but that made the curvature worsen. I also tried watsu (exercises in water with a therapist), acupuncture, osteopathic treatment, and a chiropractor. After all of those treatments proved useless, we decided to fly to Los Angeles to start treatment with a SpineCor brace. After barely a year wearing the brace, my spinal curvature had doubled. We consulted twelve different doctors in Colorado, but each one of them said that surgery was my only option. However, we kept looking for alternative treatments. We ended up overseas at Dr. Dudin's clinic. My mother and I flew to St. Petersburg, Russia, and stayed there for two months so that I could get treated. Towards the end of my treatment, I got a Chêneau brace, but it was simply unbearable. My mother and I asked where we could get a brace that was well-made, and Professor Dudin told us to go visit Dr. Weiss. This seemed like our last resort, because we were simply out of options. I got another Chêneau brace made by Mario and Peter in Bad Sobernheim, which I actually could wear, and which decreased my spinal curvature. I had to wear it for 22 hours every day, but it did not hurt me, like the previous braces. I continued going back to Germany to consult with Dr. Weiss and adjust my brace anywhere from 2-3 times a year depending on how much I had grown during that year. I ended up having 4 different braces from Dr. Weiss' clinic alone, all of which helped decrease my curvature. Dr. Weiss was always very straightforward and never promised miracles, like other doctors. He was always very kind and attentive to my needs as a patient. Thanks to Dr.Weiss' exercises and braces, I am now brace-free and surgery-free. I take dance classes and practice taekwondo. Dr. Weiss helped me to live without worries of having to get a surgery or wearing bad braces.

Thank you.

Kristina

Scoliosis Report No. 13
(AJ, 17 years, Boise, Idaho, US)

"I remember sitting in a cold room at the scoliosis specialist's office in Boise, Idaho. I had an x-ray taken of my back to measure the curve of my spine. I had to go in a room and I had to sit in front of a screen while someone turned on a light. The nurse told me to breathe in and then out. Now I realize that the reason she had me to do that was so I would sink even further in my back.

Then we went in another room to wait for the doctor. We waited for a long time until finally the doctor walked in. He started talking and what came out of his mouth was unexpected! He told us that my spine curve was 53 degrees Cobb. Above 45 Cobb degrees spine curves the only thing they do in the US was spine surgery he said. He gave us 3 websites to look at, and a YouTube with this girl's testimony about having back surgery. He said come back in 2 month to schedule the surgery.

My mom did not expect him to say this and she quickly started asking questions. Are there any other options? Could she get a brace? Maybe do physical therapy? Try anything besides surgery? The doctor said that there were absolutely no other options but surgery. He said that scoliosis couldn't reverse. It was horrible! I cried all day afterwards.

Scoliosis runs in the family, my grandma had it. My cousins, who are younger than me, also have it but not as bad. After the curve goes over 45 degrees doctors in United States only use surgery to correct it, especially if the person is still growing.

Getting a rod in my back basically meant losing all flexibility in my back, which meant that I couldn't do any sports. At the time I was in ballet and I loved it. So that was really hard to hear that I would have to give it up. After a couple very hard days, my mom and dad started researching for other ways to help reduce my curve because they were not going to let the doctors put a rod in my back.

My mom found a doctor near Frankfurt, Germany that used a traditional method, which was back bracing and physical therapy. After talking to the doctor in Germany, my parents decided to go see him that winter. My parents found out that another doctor on the East Coast took his daughter to Germany to see the same doctor and they were very happy with the results. He told my mom and dad that the doctor in Germany is the best in the world and that we will be in great hands. We couldn't be happier!

The first visit in Germany was the longest. We met Dr Weiss and his team. We had to stay there at the clinic for a whole week so they could make brace to fit my body. While I was waiting for my brace to be made I had to take some physical therapy classes and they taught me some exercises that I would have to do every day. I actually remember being excited about getting a brace, it was pretty comfortable and my back didn't hurt anymore. We went to Germany for checkups 4 times since. We loved Germany. Everybody was so nice with me. We stayed at the clinic in Gensingen and the breakfasts were delicious.

I had to wear my brace 23 hours a day, for almost 2 years. I didn't have to give up dance because Doctor Weiss said that it would actually be good for me. I was really happy that I could continue dancing. Because I had to wear it most of the day I lost a lot of flexibility in my back, which created some problems when I was dancing. Some of the teachers didn't know I had to wear it so they had very high expectations.

At first wearing the brace wasn't that bad but as soon as summer came it was really hard to get myself to wear it. I had to wear a tank top underneath it and then a shirt on top, so it got really hot. I remember that everyday at school I just wanted to go up to people and tell them to appreciate that they can wear anything they want. I always asked myself what I did to deserve this.

I'm grateful for my parents that they did everything possible to avoid surgery. I'm very thankful for Dr Weiss' dedication to get my back straight. Because I had to wear my brace 23 hours a day, and dance classes were up to three hours a day so I couldn't do any other sports. This is something I regret not being able to do the last couple of years, because ever since I was little, sports have always been an important part of my life and I had to give it up.

But the good news was that my back was getting much better. My spine curve went from 53 degrees to about 30 degrees, which meant that I didn't need surgery anymore. Last summer when I went to see the doctor again he told us that he did everything he could to help me. He was happy of how my back looked and he also told me that I could wear the brace only twelve hours a day.

This year was my first year not being in ballet, but I started playing tennis and I love it.

Today I don't have to wear my brace anymore, only sometimes at night and only if I feel I need it. My back looks straight and I measure 10-degree curve measured with the Scoliometer. Keep in mind I started at 18-degree, when I was told there is nothing that can reduce my curve!!

I don't talk about what happened because it was a really hard time for my family and me. It's really hard for me to accept that my body isn't perfect. You can still see a little bit that my back it's not straight and it will always be like this.

Even if wearing a brace 23 hours a day wasn't easy if I had a choice I will do it again. I wish more girls would choose to get the Gensingen back brace against back surgery. I'm happy my parents did all this for me and they check out different options to fix my back.

I am glad there are doctors like Dr Weiss that care about their patients and saved my back with a traditional conservative treatment. I wish other doctors in the United States would be more open to those treatments because they work.

Even though the doctor in Boise told us there is absolutely no other option to reduce a curve besides surgery, he was wrong. I can tell everybody there actually is, and I can prove it!

I wish spine doctors in America would let their patients know that surgery is NOT the only option to fix Scoliosis, and so their patients can decide what's best for them."

3 Scoliosis – What's That?

Scoliosis the term we use to refer to lateral curvature of the spine that can no longer be rectified completely *(Fig. 3.1)*. The mobility of the spinal column is reduced in the section concerned, which generally prevents the spine from being actively straightened. Such lateral curvature is combined with a twisting of the vertebral bodies, which produces the rib hump or lumbar bulge.

Scoliosis without this kind of corresponding contortion is not scoliosis in the stricter sense of the term.

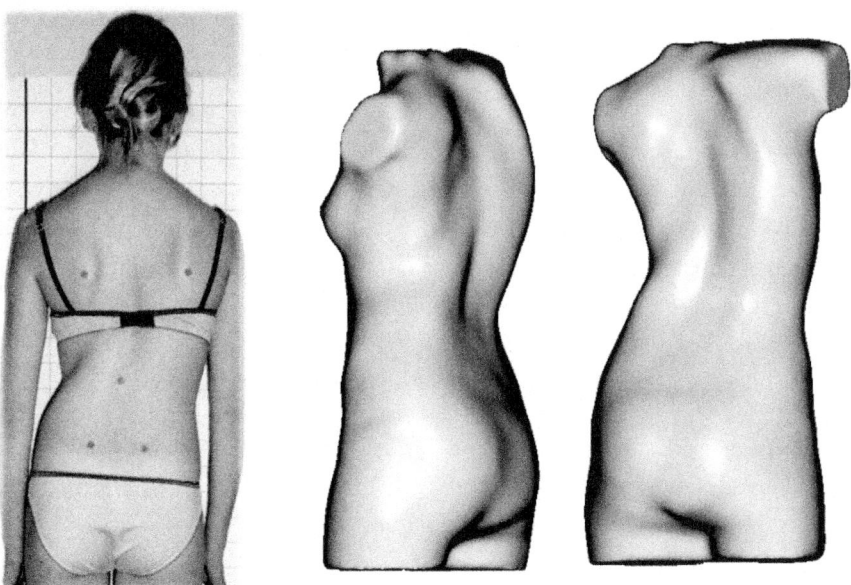

Fig. 3.1 Left: A 14-year-old female patient during a growth spurt with right-sided deviation in the thoracic area. Visible even to the layperson is the asymmetry of the waist as well as the rib hump formation on the right. The right shoulder is extended forward, with the left shoulder raised and extended backward. Since this deformity can only be minimally straightened, it meets the definition of scoliosis described as partially stiffened lateral spinal curvature. The patient in the picture has a curvature in the thoracic area of 43° measured according to Cobb. **Right:** Oblique view on a scoliosis model of the same curve pattern demonstrating the 3D deformity.

Scoliosis can have many different causes. There is scoliosis due to nerve and muscle disorders, metabolic disturbances, as well as congenital scoliosis with defective vertebral and rib development.

Most instances of scoliosis requiring treatment are due to causes not clearly defined. Despite the fact that many scientists have been endeavoring to discover the reason behind these scoliosis cases, called "idiopathic" (Lat.: arising spontaneously), not even decades of research have produced any kind of finality in this matter.

Since the majority of scoliosis patients in need of treatment have idiopathic scoliosis, for the most part I will be limiting the following discussion to this form of scoliosis.

Idiopathic scoliosis, which, incidentally, has nothing to do with the scoliosis of the suckling infant, mainly emerges during phases of increased skeleton growth.

Scoliosis occurring approximately between the first and second year of life is termed infantile idiopathic scoliosis. We call scoliosis that initially emerges between the fourth and fifth year of life juvenile idiopathic scoliosis or early onset scoliosis. Scoliosis that occurs late – between the 10th and 14th year of life – is referred to as adolescent idiopathic scoliosis or late onset scoliosis.

3.1 The Course of Untreated Idiopathic Scoliosis

The earlier idiopathic scoliosis emerges, the more unfavorable will be its anticipated course. Left untreated, early onset scoliosis (EOS) may go beyond 120 degrees, while late onset adolescent idiopathic scoliosis rarely exceeds the 90 degree limit, thus all but ruling out grave impairments to cardiovascular system function.

There are different forms of curvature, which can be roughly categorized as chest curvatures (thoracic scoliosis), lumbar curvatures (lumbar scoliosis), chest/lumbar curvatures (thoracolumbar scoliosis), or S-shaped double curvatures. Age, the onset of menstruation or voice break, signs of skeletal maturity that can be identified by the doctor on an X-ray, the severity of the curvature, gender, and the form of the curvature are considered to be the six main factors that allow doctors to assess whether the curvature can be expected to deteriorate. In girls, for example, chest curvatures with a right rib hump are statistically more likely to become increasingly pronounced than are double curvatures with a right rib hump. Furthermore, it can be assumed that the risk for curvature increase is greater in younger patients than in nearly mature individuals. This is quite understandable if we bear in mind that – in phases of more rapid spinal growth – vertebrae with a wedge shape will continue to mature wedge-shaped, since they are put under stress and strain asymmetrically. When growth is complete, such speedy deterioration is no longer possible.

According to a recent review[1] late onset idiopathic scoliosis (Adolescent Idiopathic Scoliosis) can be regarded as being benign, although in some presentations spine surgeons tend to dramatize this kind of scoliosis.

3.2 The Course of Treated Idiopathic Scoliosis

Danielsson and collaborators have compiled the long-term results of scoliosis treatment with brace and operation.[2] According to these study results, both surgically as well as non-surgically treated scoliosis patients must expect to suffer considerable mobility restrictions, a generally poorer state of health, and somewhat more pain than people without scoliosis. The last of the three stands in direct contrast to earlier studies, according to which scoliosis patients do not have to anticipate an increased incidence of pain. Since the authors have not been able to discover any crucial differences between surgically and non-surgically treated scoliosis patients with regard to health-related adverse effects, this begs the question as to whether an operation leads to an improvement in the state of health of scoliosis patients or not.

In the Oswestry Disability Questionnaire, a questionnaire to assess physical and social restrictions, there were marked differences between the scoliosis

---

[1] Weiss HR, Karavidas N, Moramarco M, Moramarco K: Long-term effects of untreated Adolescent Idiopathic Scoliosis – Review of the literature. Asian Spine Journal, in press.
[2] Danielsson AJ, Wiklund I, Pehrsson K, Nachemson AL (2001) Health-related quality of life in patients with adolescent idiopathic scoliosis: a matched follow-up at least 20 years after treatment with brace or surgery. Eur Spine J 10:278–288

patients studied and a control group without scoliosis. The two test groups – surgically and non-surgically treated scoliosis patients – had functional limitations compared to the control group without scoliosis.

Both surgically as well as conservatively treated scoliosis patients had adverse effects as far as their social activities were concerned, with the patients who had been operated on comparatively less able to participate in sporting activities. This test group also indicated an increased fear of being injured.

There are greater signs of wear or degeneration visible on an X-ray in the treated scoliosis patients than in the control group without scoliosis, but the frequency is the same in surgically and conservatively treated scoliosis patients.[3]

Differences in the lung or pulmonary function were not found in surgically and conservatively treated scoliosis patients with adolescent idiopathic scoliosis.

In cases of adolescent idiopathic scoliosis, those affected mainly had misgivings about their appearance. Since it is well known that this form of scoliosis does not have any serious health implications, this may not be much of surprise to anyone. We also know that a scoliosis operation does not have a favorable influence on the health of those afflicted and is therefore ruled out for health reasons alone.[4] Even the cosmetic improvements after an operation are not always stable.[3,5]

Due to the fact that a rib hump may recur worse than before within 12 months of the operation,[4] and the long-term surgical risks are not

---

[3] Danielsson AJ, Nachemson AL (2001) Radiologic Findings and Curve Progression 22 Years After Treatment for Adolescent Idiopathic Scoliosis. Spine 26 (5):516–552

[4] Hawes M. Impact of spine surgery on signs and symptoms of spinal deformity. Pediatr Rehabil. 2006 Oct-Dec; 9(4):318–39.

[5] Weiss HR, Bess S, Wong MS, Patel V, Goodall D, Burger E. Adolescent idiopathic scoliosis - to operate or not? A debate article. Patient Saf Surg. 2008 Sep 30;2(1):25.

foreseeable,[6] the low-risk option of providing a suitable brace to improve the appearance should be attempted. After all, significant cosmetic improvements can also be attained with cutting-edge brace strategies.[7] As to whether these strategies remain stable in the long term, however, is unknown – just as with operations.

Recent systematic reviews and a Cochrane review clearly show that according to the current scientific literature there is no evidence that would support spinal fusion surgery.[8,9]

Health related signs and symptoms of a scoliosis obviously are not influenced by spinal fusion surgery[4,8,9,10], therefore evidence based high quality conservative measures must be applied primarily.

---

[6] Weiss HR, Goodall D. Rate of complications in scoliosis surgery - a systematic review of the Pub Med literature. Scoliosis. 2008 Aug 5;3:9.
[7] Weiss HR, Moramarco M. Remodeling of trunk and backshape deformities in patients with scoliosis using standardized asymmetric CAD / CAM braces. Hard Tissue 2013 Feb 26;2(2):14.
[8] Bettany-Saltikov J, Weiss HR, Chockalingam N, Taranu R, Srinivas S, Hogg J, et al. Surgical versus non-surgical interventions in people with adolescent idiopathic scoliosis. Cochrane Database Syst Rev. 2015;4:CD010663.
[9] Westrick E, Ward W. Adolescent idiopathic scoliosis: 5-year to 20-year evidence-based surgical results. J Pediatr Orthop. 2011;31(1 Suppl):S61 - S8.
[10] Ward WT RJ, Friel N, Kenkre TS, Brooks MM SRS 22r Scores in Non-Operated AIS Patients with Curves ≥ 40°. Proceedings of the 50th Annual Meeting Minneapolis, Minnesota, US, 2015, September 30th – October 3rd. 2015.

4 What Has to Be Measured?

The attending physician requires certain measuring procedures to be able to control the course of the spinal curvature. He has to be able to assess in the early phase whether a case of scoliosis solely meriting observation to date has deteriorated to such a degree that treatment is necessary. When scoliosis needs treatment, he must be able to discern whether physical therapy is sufficient or whether providing a brace and pattern specific rehabilitation will be required. For scoliosis treated with a brace, he has to determine whether the curvature is increasing despite the use of the brace. This, as well as the difficulties in predicting the course means it makes sense to have a medical checkup every quarter, perhaps with longer intervals during slower growth phases.

The attending physician uses measuring procedures that allow for comparisons to be made at a later date.

So what needs to be measured?

4.1 Radiography

In order to diagnose scoliosis, the doctor needs an X-ray. Where possible, a standing full spinal X-ray *(Fig. 4.1)* should be made to monitor the course of the condition and be taken from either the front or the back as well as from the side. The frontal X-ray can be used to measure the angle of curvature and identify whether there are any rib or spinal deformities. This will, for instance, verify the diagnosis of idiopathic scoliosis or – in cases where there are spinal or rib deformities – the diagnosis of congenital scoliosis. The lateral X-ray allows for any spinal deformities in this plane or for hollow-back in the area of the thoracic spine to be detected. Such a case of hollow-back is of significance when deriving a prognosis.

X-rays of this kind and size naturally entail a certain amount of radiation exposure. However, this cannot be avoided. X-rays are essential any time that deterioration is anticipated after clinical measurements have been taken or even for monitoring brace treatment.

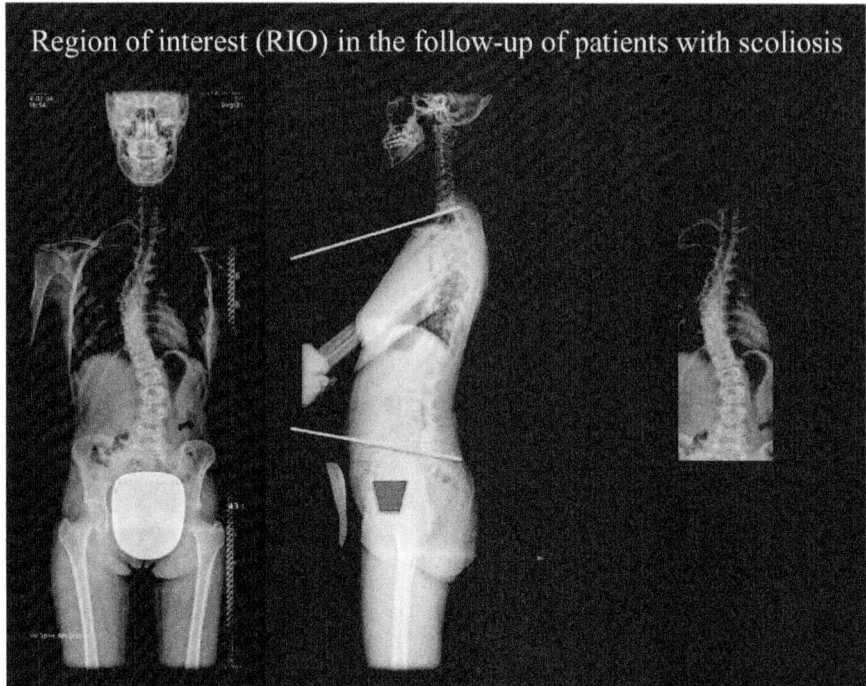

Fig. 4.1: Image of the entire spinal column of a patient with idiopathic scoliosis. As can be seen the head and parts of the legs are on the x-ray which is not necessary at all. On the side view (*middle* picture) there is no shelter applied. On the *right* picture one can see the region of interest (ROI) allowing to diagnose the patient well and to measure the Cobb angle. Exposure to radiation drastically can be reduced by limiting the field to the ROI.[11]

However, after the initial X-ray assessment the author does not even regularly order a lateral view since, for conservative treatment, the lateral profile of the spine can be determined sufficiently using clinical methods.

Furthermore, taking a so-called "low-dose" X-ray enables the radiation dose to be reduced by shortening the exposure time accordingly, provided that it is only a matter of measuring the angle of curvature. Unfortunately, this kind of radiation-saving image is only suitable for patients who do not have excessive fat deposits.

---

[11] Weiss HR, Seibel S: Region of Interest (ROI) in the radiological follow-up of patients with scoliosis Hard Tissue 2: 2013;33. June.

The orthopedist uses the X-ray to measure the angle of curvature, generally according to Cobb *(Figs. 4.2 and 4.3)*. This angle of curvature is also checked in the follow-up X-rays. The treatment guidelines can then be deduced from the size of this angle.

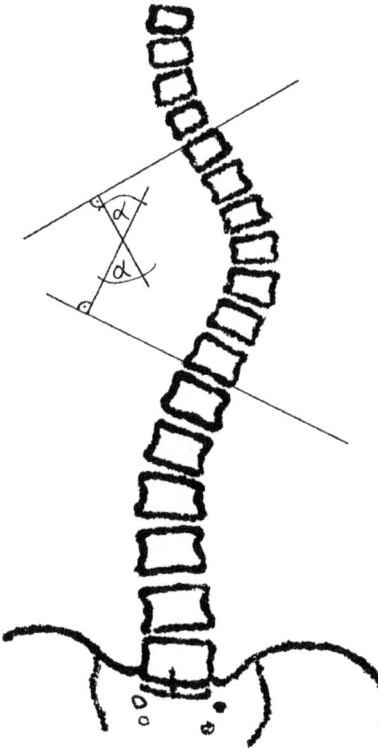

Fig. 4.2: Schematic representation of the curvature angle formation. The plate covering the upper neutral vertebra, which generally is tilted the most, has been marked with a tangent line, as has the end plate of the lower neutral vertebra. Vertical lines (on the left side of the image here) are aligned with these tangents, crossing to form the curvature angle according to Cobb (labeled here with the angle symbol).

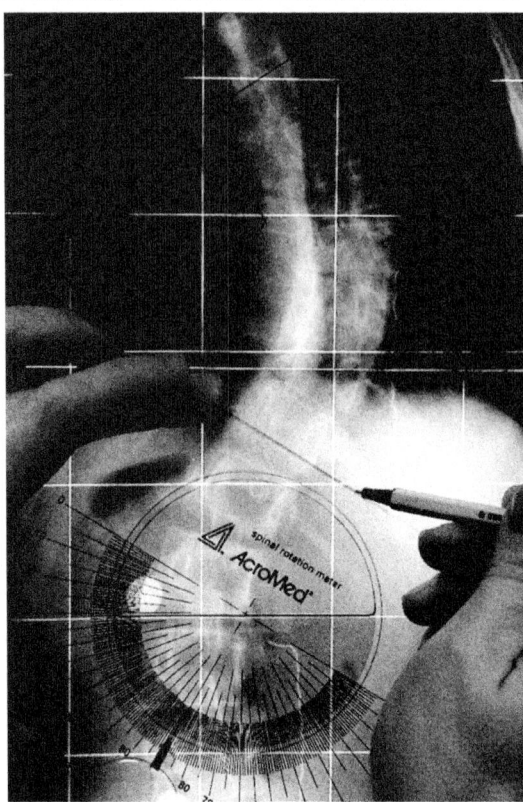

Fig. 4.3: The Cobb angle can also be derived with the help of a device that allows the tilt of the neutral vertebrae to be determined.

Recently a new stereo radiographic system has been released. The EOS Imaging System is a full body low dose system allowing a 3D reconstruction of the spine and an automated objective measurement of kyphosis and scoliosis (Cobb) angles. There is access to the images (Fig 4.4) and also to the comprehensive report (Fig 4.5) which is automatically recorded.

The disadvantage of the system currently is the high acquisition cost.

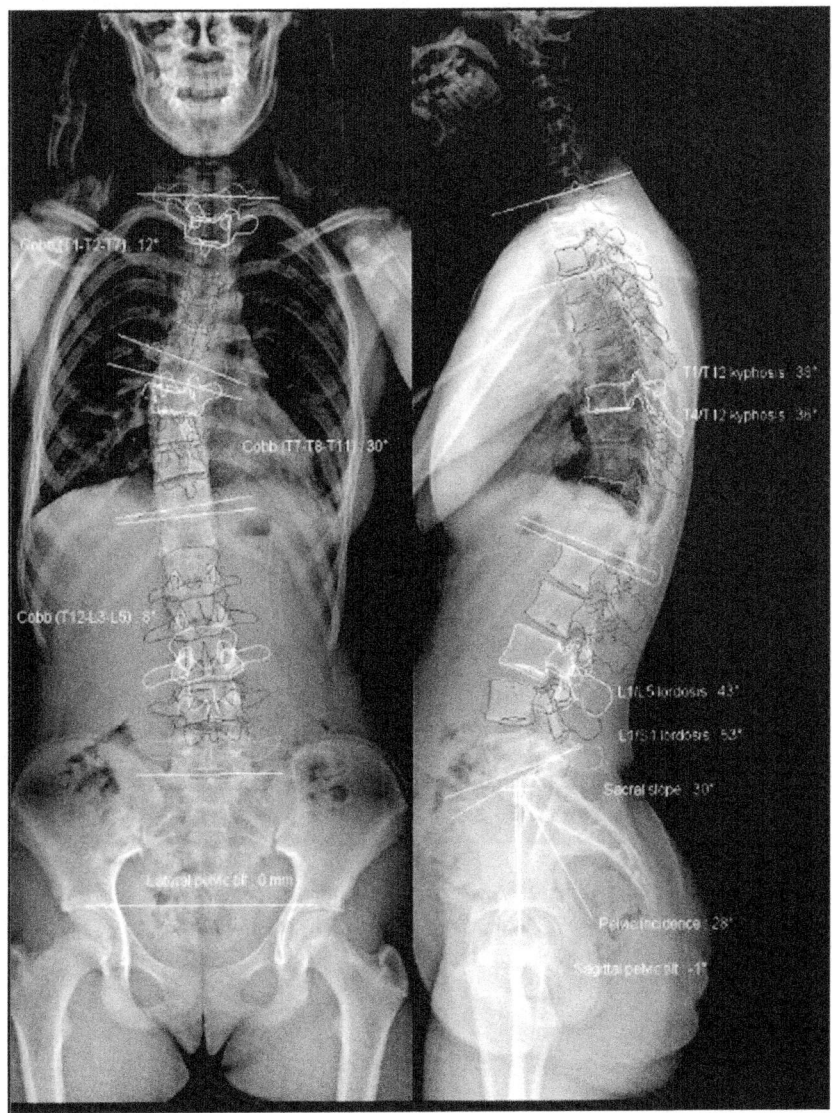

Fig. 4.4: Images from an EOS system with automated calculations of the angles of curvature (with kind permission by Daniel Comerford, Melbourne).

56 | Chapter 4. What Has to Be Measured?

Spine parameters			
Scoliosis parameters (1)		Value	
Curve (T6-T8-T10)	Cobb (T6-T8-T10)	19°	
	Axial rotation of apical vertebra T8	11°	
Curve (T11-L1-L3)	Cobb (T11-L1-L3)	16°	
	Axial rotation of apical vertebra L1	12°	
Sagittal balance (1)		Value	
T1/T12 kyphosis		39°	
T4/T12 kyphosis		35°	
L1/L5 lordosis		39°	
L1/S1 lordosis		40°	

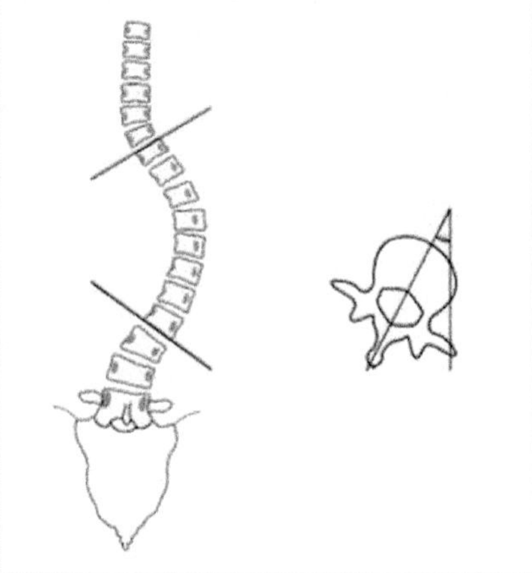

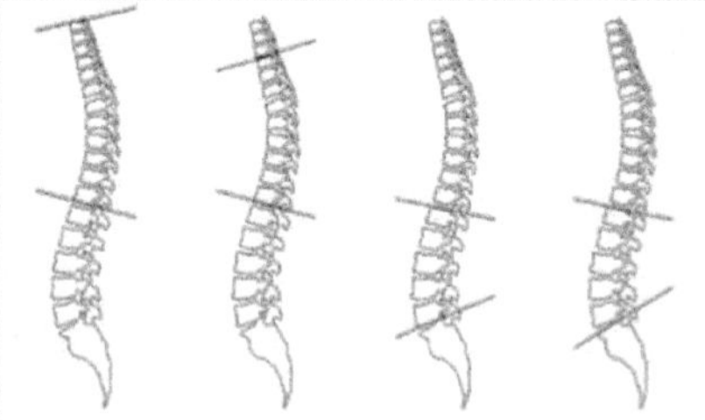

(1) Parameters calculated in the patient frame (based on a vertical plane passing through the center of the cotyles), which corrects the effect of a potential axial rotation of the pelvis during acquisition.
An axial vertebra rotation is positive when the vertebra is rotated towards the patient left side.

Fig 4.5: Part of the EOS Imaging report (with kind permission by Daniel Comerford, Melbourne).

4.2 Clinical Measuring Procedures

The clinical measuring procedures used include: determining body size when standing as well as when sitting, body weight, and also respiratory volume – quite different measured values, which, however, are not always routinely carried out in practice.

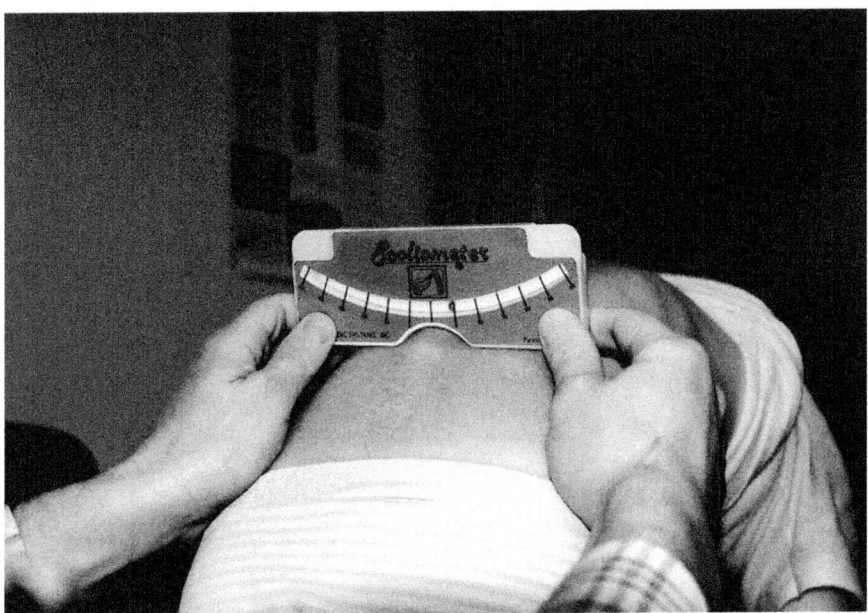

Fig. 4.6: Measuring the lumbar bulge (hump) with the scoliometer according to Bunnel in an Adams forward bending test.

It is important for practical use to have clinical measuring procedures that enable curvature values to be compared directly. The simplest measuring procedure in this context is measuring trunk asymmetry with the Scoliometer according to Bunnel *(Fig. 4.6)*. This was developed in the USA, primarily for the purpose of providing a simple and inexpensive measuring method for screening exams in schools. However, this measuring instrument should also be available in orthopedic practices that deal with scoliosis, since it can be used during checkups to pinpoint significant indications of possible curvature deterioration. Scoliometer measurement (angle of trunk rotation – ATR) is performed during the Adams forward bending test with knees in extension. Any pelvic obliquity must be counteracted beforehand. Such differences in leg length may sometimes change in quarterly intervals in children and adolescents who are still growing, which is why they need to be accounted for in the measurement.

When this Scoliometer measurement is taken by the same doctor on each visit, it is very significant and a low repetitive error rate of approximately 1 to 1.5 degrees.

4.3 Surface Topography

Since scoliosis is initially conspicuous due to a change in the shape of the back, it is conceivable that this changed back shape could be photographed and then perhaps evaluated with a computer. The use of surface topography systems is becoming more and more widespread. Such topography systems not only make it possible to store the shape of the back on the computer and print out the computer image, but also to automatically determine a multitude of measurement data and make them available for subsequent comparison.

In times past, scoliosis children were X-rayed about four times a year, leading to high radiation exposure. The availability of the surface topography procedure makes it possible to do without an X-ray examination for as long as there is no indication that deterioration has occurred. Radiation doses can thus be reduced, in hopes of lowering the demonstratably increased risk borne by scoliosis patients from being repeatedly exposed to radiation.

Various measuring procedures are available for monitoring the course of spinal curvatures.

The QUANTEC and ISIS systems produced in England have been especially designed for scoliosis progress monitoring. Since these measuring instruments are unable to calculate scoliosis unless marking tape is affixed, they have less measurement accuracy compared to fully automated equipment such as the FORMETRIC system developed in Germany.

The FORMETRIC system recognizes the back topography automatically, calculating the curvature from the coordinates it has determined. It provides a large number of measurement data automatically as well *(Fig. 4.7)*. Not only can it ascertain scoliosis of the spine, but also humpback and hollow-back. (This allows for the course of posture disorders and kyphosis to be monitored too.)

The FORMETRIC system is therefore accurate enough to take the place of X-rays at least some of the time. Should the findings indicate that deterioration has taken place, however, an X-ray examination will be indispensable – the same as when checking treatment using a brace. The natural shifting of posture during measuring prevents the measured values describing scolioses from being very exact. A technical error lying between 15 and 20% of the measurement result is definitely too imprecise for comparative analysis. It is true, however, that the specialist may well obtain additional information by comparing images.

In contrast, the measurement results for kyphosis (humpback) can be compared exceedingly well. The lateral view of the spinal curvature can therefore be documented and analyzed without an X-ray examination.

There has recently been an increasing amount of scientific evidence pointing to the fact that the lateral view of the spinal curvature pattern is of great significance with respect to the occurrence of chronic back pain. In particular, it seems that reducing thoracic hollow-back or lumbar kyphosis directly affects back pain. This is the reason why surface topography will be playing a greater role in the future in the areas of progress monitoring and treating pain.

Now the spine can also be measured dynamically on the treadmill. This makes it possible for asymmetrical movement patterns to be recognized and corrected (see: Scoliologic® 'Best Practice' Programm[12,13,14]).

---

[12] Weiss HR, Seibel S (2010). Scoliosis Short-Term Rehabilitation (SSTR) – A Pilot Investigation, The Internet Journal of Rehabilitation. 1: 1. 11

[13] Borysov M, Borysov A. Scoliosis short-term rehabilitation (SSTR) according to 'Best Practice' standards-are the results repeatable? Scoliosis. 2012 Jan 17;7(1):1. doi: 10.1186/1748-7161-7-1.

[14] Pugacheva N. Corrective exercises in multimodality therapy of idiopathic scoliosis in children - analysis of six weeks efficiency - pilot study. Stud Health Technol Inform. 2012;176:365-71.

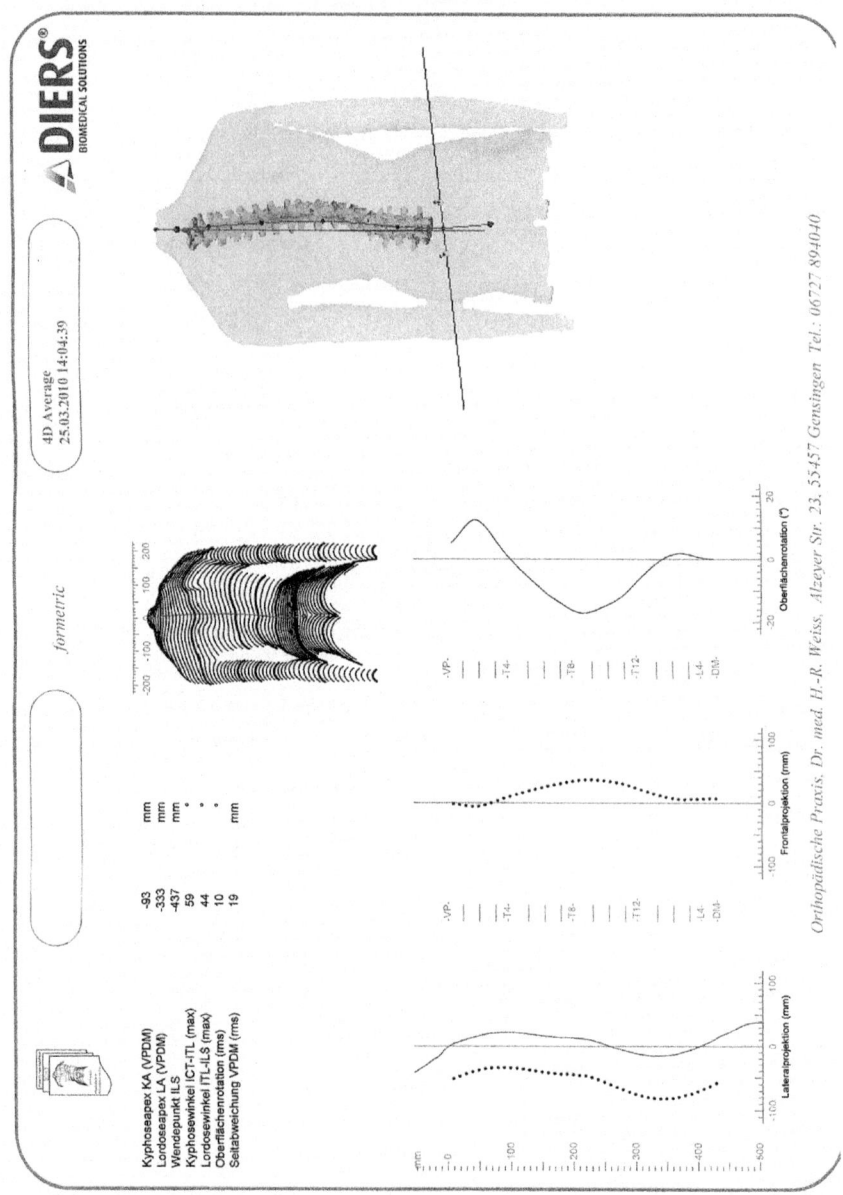

Fig. 4.7: Printout of the cover page of a surface survey carried out with the Formetric system. At the top right, the profile lines graphically illustrating the extent of the spinal curvature are visible. To the left, a long row of measured values for monitoring the progression can be seen.

Tests with 3D whole-body scanners, used for trunk measurement in preparation for a brace, are the very latest development. When using these scanners for suitable measured values, clinical progress monitoring can be conducted at the same time that the patient's measurements needed for providing a brace are obtained. In the future, such multifunction use may well enable specialist practices to offer surface topography for monitoring patients with spinal deformities to members of statutory health insurance companies at more affordable prices.

5 Treatment

What does scoliosis treatment consist of and why does such treatment have to be done at all?

In the case of minor curvatures, treatment is primarily intended to prevent them from growing any larger; for major curvatures, the intent is to alleviate the consequences of scoliosis. A scoliosis operation is intended to improve the patient's appearance and potential function and to serve as a deterrent against further deterioration of the condition. Certainly, Feldenkrais, Eutony, Osteopathy, Qigong or acupressure may well be a useful and beneficial supplement in individual cases. However, none of these measures should be allowed to take the place of the verifiably effective treatment strategies described below.

5.1 Physical Rehabilitation

Particularly in Germany, there is quite a long tradition of using physical therapy to treat scoliosis. As early as the beginning of the 19th century, institutes were opened at various locations in Germany that sought to improve the posture of patients in their care under inpatient conditions. Before the turn of the 20th century, a whole array of equipment was employed for scoliosis treatment that was supposed to flatten the rib hump or fortify the trunk muscles. At the beginning of the century, scoliosis was combated using methods that included "KLAPP crawling," while the introduction of "three-dimensional scoliosis treatment according to Katharina SCHROTH" in 1921 marked the first time that the hitherto purely mechanical approach to treatment was abandoned in favor of more holistically oriented treatment.[15,16] In the last century, several physiotherapeutic procedures for treating scoliosis were described that, for the most part, are hardly taught anymore today and have therefore all but

---

[15] Lehnert-Schroth Ch (2000) Dreidimensionale Skoliosebehandlung, 6th ed., Urban und Fischer

[16] Weiß HR (2011) Befundgerechte Physiotherapie bei Skoliose, 3rd ed., Pflaum Verlag

disappeared. What has been scientifically investigated are both three-dimensional scoliosis treatment according to Katharina SCHROTH and developmental kinesiology treatment according to VOJTA. In addition to three-dimensional scoliosis treatment according to Katharina SCHROTH, the Side Shift program is also known internationally as a specific treatment measure, besides non-specific treatments like Yoga, DoboMed, and SEAS.

While patients receiving treatment according to VOJTA *(Fig. 5.1)* are dependent on a therapist, help for self-help stands at the forefront of three-dimensional scoliosis treatment according to Katharina SCHROTH *(Fig. 5.2)*. For this reason, the treatment method according to VOJTA is recommended more for patients with smaller curvatures and at younger ages, while scoliosis treatment according to K. SCHROTH is more important after age 10 as well as for adult patients.

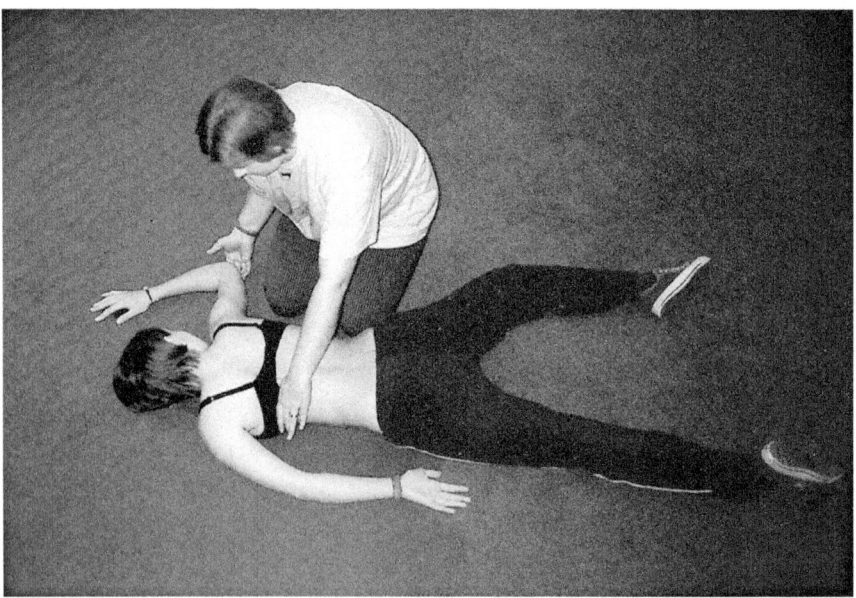

Fig. 5.1: Exercise for facilitating so-called reflex creeping from the exercise program according to Vojta.

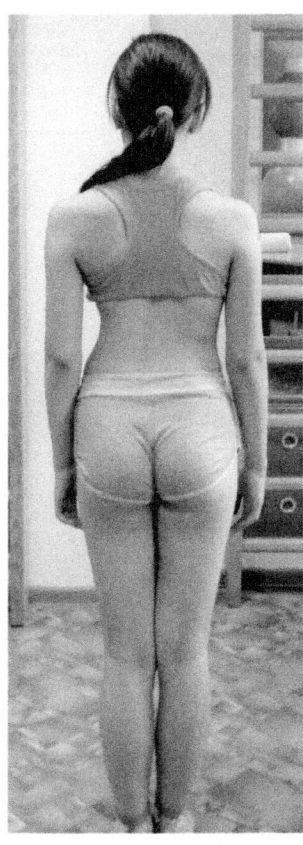 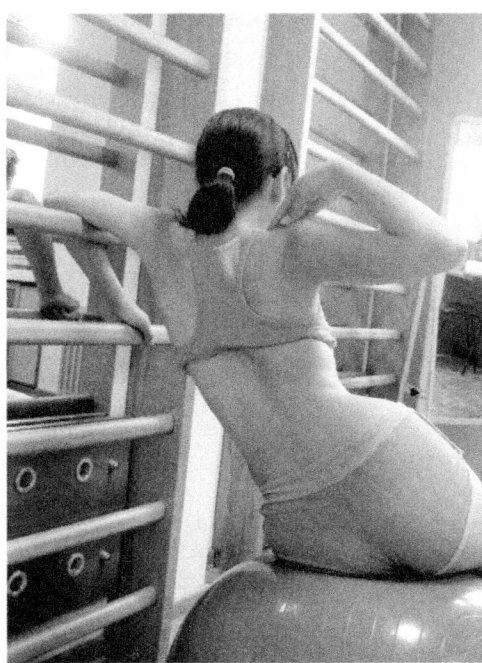

Figs. 5.2 Left: Female scoliosis patient with a right thoracic scoliosis, right-sided rib hump, and a right-sided deviation in the thoracic area when at rest. **Right:** Exercise from the 'Best Practice' program as derived from the three-dimensional scoliosis treatment program according to Katharina-Schroth. It can be clearly seen here how the right-sided deviation is rebalanced and even the rib hump reduced with the help of breathing during the exercise (Borysov and Borysov *Scoliosis* 2012 **7**:1).

There are still other methods of physiotherapeutic scoliosis treatment practiced outside of Germany that are not as widespread. However, applying general treatment procedures not specifically developed for scoliosis flies in the face of scientific findings that have since been obtained concerning the efficacy of such special methods as Schroth, Schroth Best Practice, and Side Shift.

The effectiveness of intensive physiotherapeutic measures has already been described in various studies. It can be concluded from these studies that scoliosis can be corrected in certain cases by physical therapy and that the burden of wearing a brace can be considerably lessened by physiotherapeutic treatment.

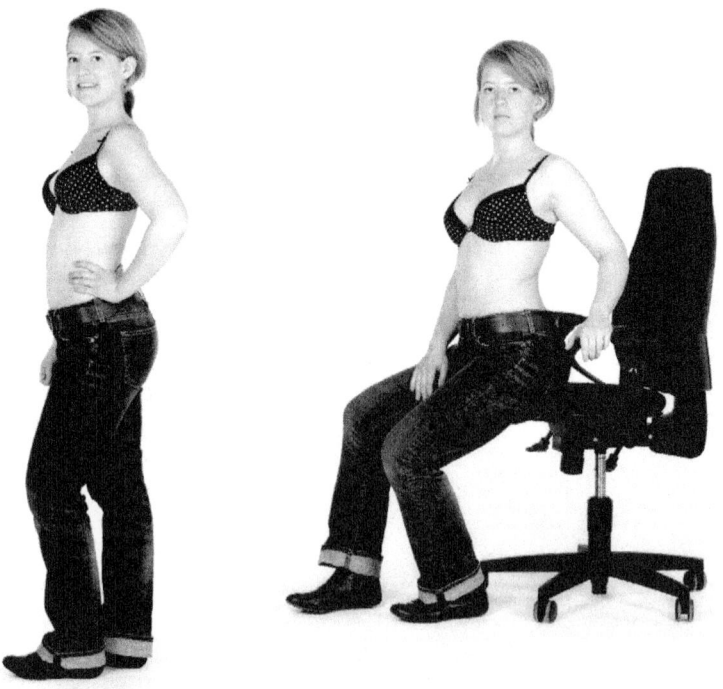

Fig. 5.3: Everyday postures from the physio-logic® program in standing and seated position.

More recent scientific findings concerning the correctibility of scoliosis arrive at the conclusion that spinal scoliosis as well as spinal rotation can be reduced by a simple corrective movement. A reduction in outwardly visible scoliosis phenomena is possible by merely increasing the hollow-back (lordosis) at the level of the 1st lumbar vertebra in conjunction with increasing the humpback (kyphosis) in the lower thoracic area. As a consequence of this, exercises for strengthening the lateral profile (sagittal profile) have recently been integrated more and more into the Schroth concept *(Fig. 5.3)*. Corresponding exercises can be carried out on wall bars as well as in a hallway *(Figs. 5.4)*.

5.1 Physical Rehabilitation | 67

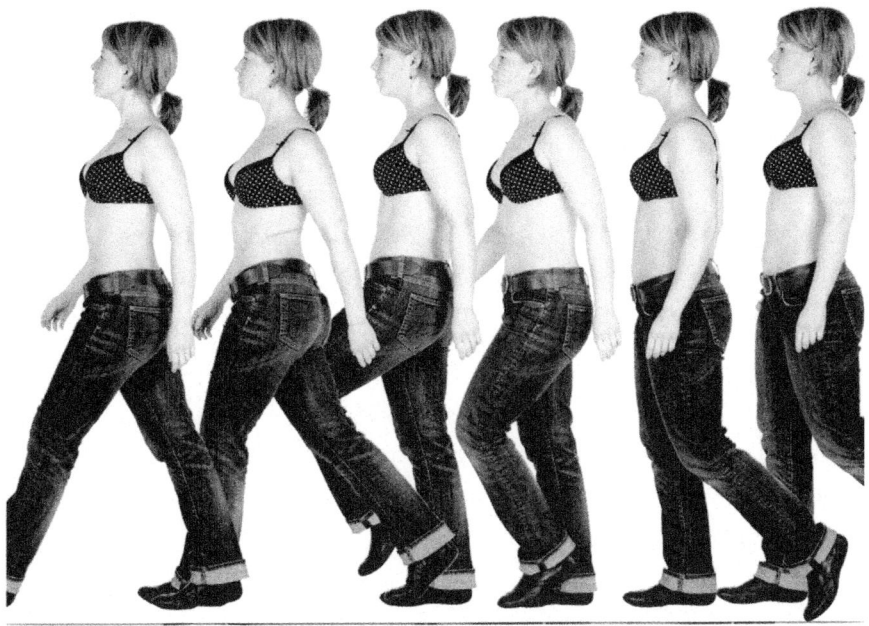

Figs. 5.4: The so-called "catwalk" allows for good mobilization with a relatively normal lateral profile if the lower costal arch can rock forward along with the step rhythm.

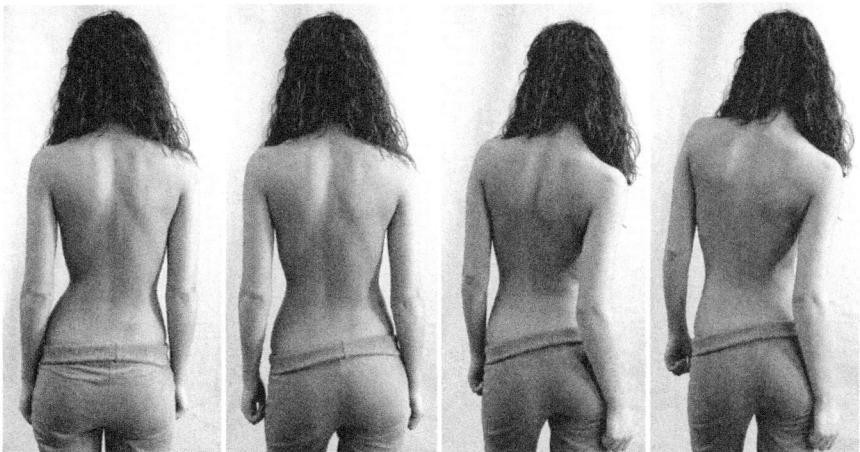

Fig. 5.5: Four-step exercise sequence from the "3D Made Easy" program for functional three-curve scoliosis: 1. Position the pelvis in the opposite direction; 2. correct the shoulder girdle; 3. breathe in using the left thoracic area; and 4. stabilize.

Simpler treatment techniques, such as "3D exercises made easy," have been developed of late. As can be seen on *Figure 5.5* for a functional triple curve, this new treatment technique is applied accordingly to the individual curvature pattern.

These new ways of treatment are also being applied in more modern rehabilitation concepts that increasingly need to adapt to the fact that patients can no longer miss six weeks of school without the risk of being put at a disadvantage.

As a matter of fact exercises performed for 20 minutes each day will not be sufficient to influence the course of scoliosis at large. Therefore, activities of daily living (ADLs) have recently gained importance. A full day self-management is possible once the curvature pattern specific ADLs are applied in everyday life *(Fig. 5.6)*.

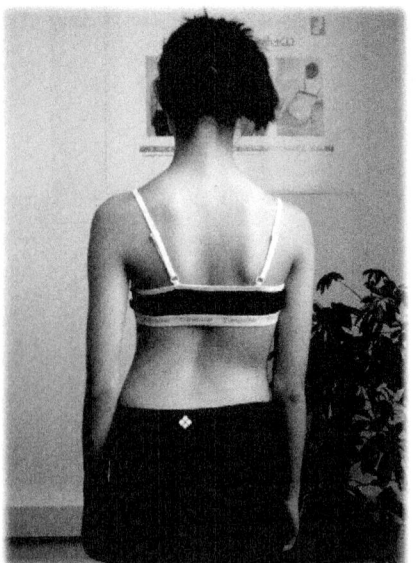 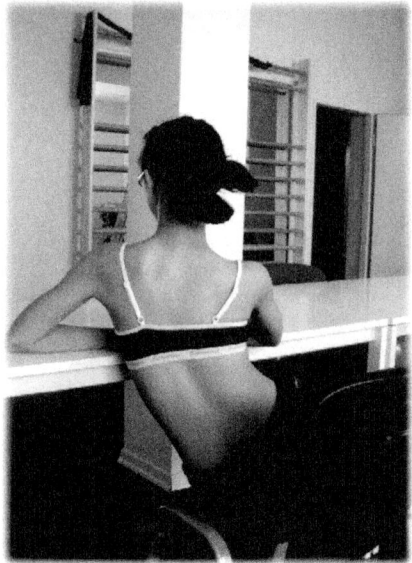

Fig. 5.6: "Wipe your neighbor away from the table!" The patient (pattern 3CH, still very flexible) can completely correct her curvature using this exercise from the *ADL* program. The right hip can move upwards. The patient therefore crosses her right leg (the leg on the costal hump side) over the left leg. For pattern 4C, the left leg (the leg on the costal cavity side) must be crossed over the right leg in order to prevent the right hip from moving upward. In doing so, a worsening of the lumbar countercurve can be prevented.

However, group treatment for scoliosis patients works especially well, since those afflicted do not feel so alone with their problems, and an exchange of experiences can take place that provides emotional release.

A Cochrane review supports the use of physiotherapy in the management of scoliosis.[17]

Meanwhile there are three randomized controlled studies on corrective exercises,[18-20] however only the paper by Kuru et al.[20] provided an untreated control group. Kuru et al.[20] have tested the recent Schroth Best Practice concept and compared the results achieved with a group of scoliosis patients receiving no treatment.

5.2 Brace Treatment

The efficacy of wearing a brace has likewise been borne out by a multitude of studies and is supported by a Cochrane review. Wearing a brace is thus an effective, albeit involved treatment, which has to be carefully planned and carried out. When making braces, it is the experience of the orthopedic technician that is of decisive importance, while brace acceptance naturally depends on the experience of the attending physician. For this reason, such treatment should only be reserved for a treatment team that provides at least 50 scoliosis patients a year with braces or that is under guidance of an experienced specialist. There is a dependent correlation between the end result and both the corrective effect and wearing time. The technician and

---

[17] Romano M, Minozzi S, Bettany-Saltikov J, Zaina F, Chockalingam N, Kotwicki T, et al. Exercises for adolescent idiopathic scoliosis. *Cochrane Database Syst Rev.* 2012;8.

[18] Monticone M, Ambrosini E, Cazzaniga D, Rocca B, Ferrante S. Active self-correction and task-oriented exercises reduce spinal deformity and improve quality of life in subjects with mild adolescent idiopathic scoliosis. Results of a randomised controlled trial. *Eur Spine J.* 2014;23(6):1204-14.

[19] Schreiber S, Parent EC, Moez EK, Hedden DM, Hill D, Moreau MJ, et al. The effect of Schroth exercises added to the standard of care on the quality of life and muscle endurance in adolescents with idiopathic scoliosis-an assessor and statistician blinded randomized controlled trial: "SOSORT 2015 Award Winner". *Scoliosis.* 2015;10:24.

[20] Kuru T, Yeldan I, Dereli EE, Ozdincler AR, Dikici F, Colak I. The efficacy of three-dimensional Schroth exercises in adolescent idiopathic scoliosis: a randomised controlled clinical trial. *Clin Rehabil.* 2016;30:181-190.

doctor must ensure a good corrective effect and wearability, with the patients themselves seeing to the proper wearing time.

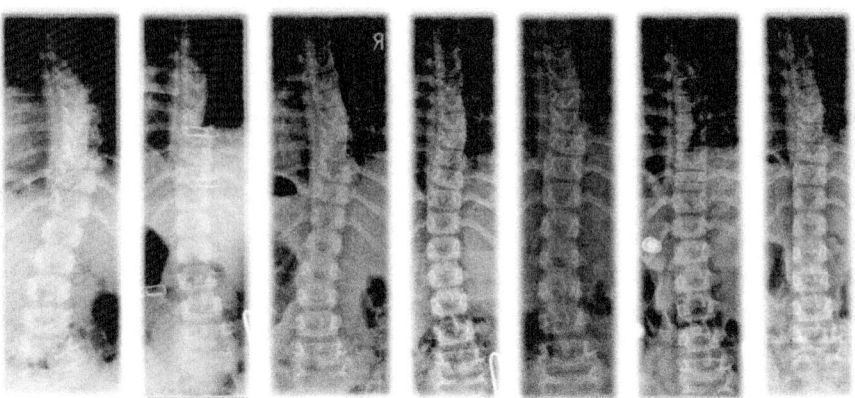

Fig. 5.7: Progression of juvenile idiopathic scoliosis (early onset scoliosis) with a curvature angle of more than 30° at age 6. A continuous reduction in the curvature was attained by constantly wearing a CAD Chêneau brace brace for approx. 16 hours a day. She entered the pubertal growth spurt with less than 20° and therefore only required a wearing time of 12 hours/day during the main growth spurt.

Wearing a brace is necessary if it is suspected that physiotherapeutic measures alone will not be sufficient. We can assume this in the following cases:

1. Even before physical maturity is reached when a child is with the first signs of maturation, the angle of curvature is at 20 degrees. While it is true that in 8 to 10% of the cases, scoliosis may spontaneously remit, this only affects slight curvatures of less than 20 degrees in children who are not yet mature. As of 20 degrees of curvature, it unfortunately has to be assumed that scoliosis will progress unfavorably once those afflicted enter the main growth spurt. During this phase of life, drastic deterioration in scoliosis may occur within a matter of a few weeks (more than 20 degrees a year), making growth-channeling measures necessary. It is not uncommon that scoliosis with relatively slight curvatures (20 to 30 degrees) can be largely corrected at this age *(Fig. 5.7)* or even overcorrected, meaning that regularly wearing of a properly made orthosis can result in significant final corrections or even – in rare cases – complete curvature straightening after

the patient has been weaned off the brace. In other words, sometimes there is the chance to take advantage of a growth spurt to straighten a curvature that would get worse without a brace. Once menstruation or voice break have set in, the peak of the growth rate is generally past and sustained curvature straightening can no longer be expected.

2. A curvature in excess of 20 degrees deteriorates by more than five degrees after the menstruation or voice break have occured. Even then the scoliosis is to be categorized as progressive, and so wearing a brace to safeguard against expected growth is indicated.

3. Wearing a brace is effective up to one year after the onset of menstruation if the angle of curvature is more than 30 degrees. In cases of delayed bone maturity and curvatures over 40 degrees, it is often advisable even through the end of the second year after the onset of menstruation.

Three year follow-up

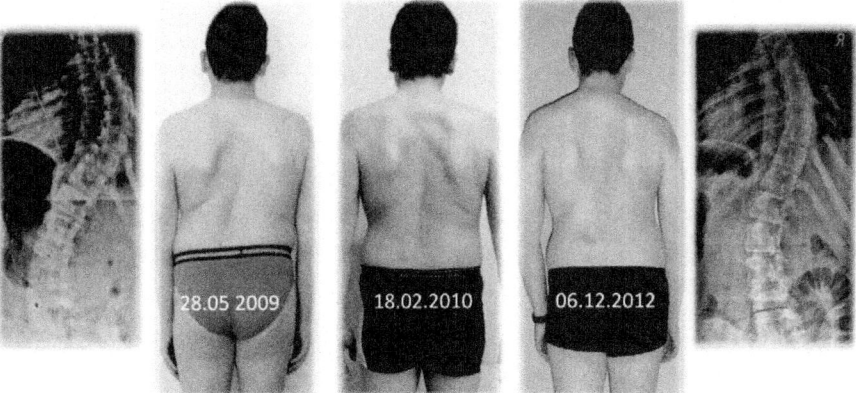

Fig. 5.8: Progression of adolescent idiopathic scoliosis in an adolescent boy with a curvature of 56° at the beginning of treatment. Afterwards, the curvature in the X-ray is reduced, markedly compensated, and clinically all but invisible. (From: *Weiss HR, Moramarco M. Remodeling of trunk and backshape deformities in patients with scoliosis using standardized asymmetric CAD / CAM braces. Hard Tissue 2013 Feb 26;2(2):14.*)

It was hitherto assumed that braces can only be effective up to an angle of curvature of 40 degrees. However, even beyond this limit, there are favorable outcomes by using brace treatment *(Fig. 5.8)*. Especially against the backdrop of it being only a relative necessity for operating on adolescent idiopathic scoliosis – only when there are rather severe psychological problems due to cosmetic changes, really – brace treatment increases in importance even for greater curvatures. It has been shown that there is no increased risk, whether in patients with adolescent idiopathic scoliosis or with late onset scoliosis of unknown origin, of coming down with severe cardiopulmonary problems, especially because a curvature of 80 to 90 degrees is practically never attained.

It is only beyond this limit that serious problems due to lung function impairment are expected. Furthermore, with late onset scoliosis (initial onset at an age between the 10th and 14th year of life), it is indicated there is essentially no increased susceptibility to pain in comparison to a control group of adults not affected by scoliosis. For this reason, an operation in this group is only necessary if the spinal curvature causes immense psychological strain. There is a real chance to achieve clinical corrections comparable to the ones after surgery when braces according to the highest standards are applied *(Fig. 5.9 and 5.10)*.

Providing scoliosis patients with braces is a responsible task of specialized orthopedists and orthopedic technicians that generally, when properly carried out, is not only able to prevent further trunk deformity, but also facilitates significant cosmetic improvements when there is still residual growth. Such improvements can only be achieved, however, if three-dimensional trunk deformity with scoliosis is accounted for in an optimum manner.

Many treatment concepts using braces (trunk orthoses) are currently being pursued, most of them with slight to moderate treatment success. Orthopedic technicians, who make good corrective effects possible with bracing, are not available everywhere.

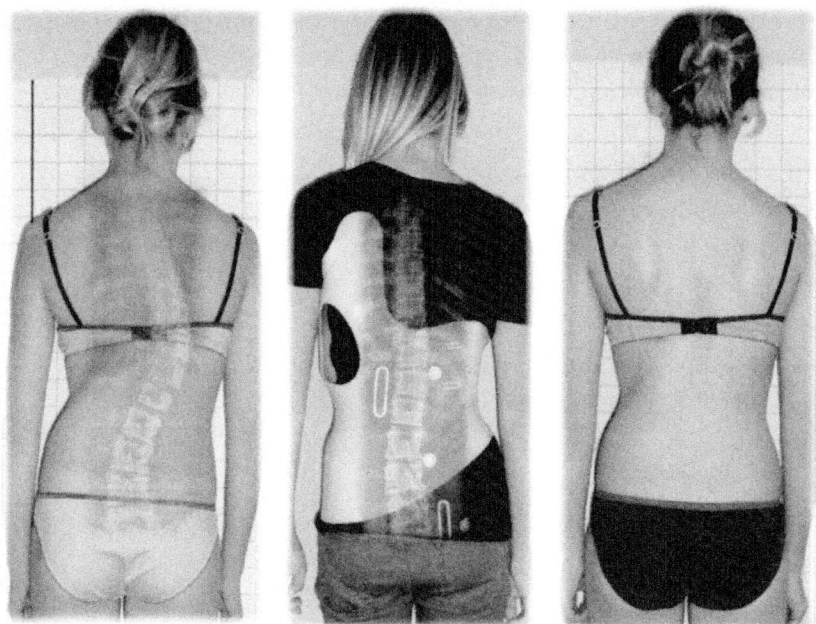

Fig. 5.9: Girl with a right thoracic curve of 42° treated in a CAD / CAM Chêneau brace of the Gensingen library with an intermediate correction in frontal plane as visible on the right.

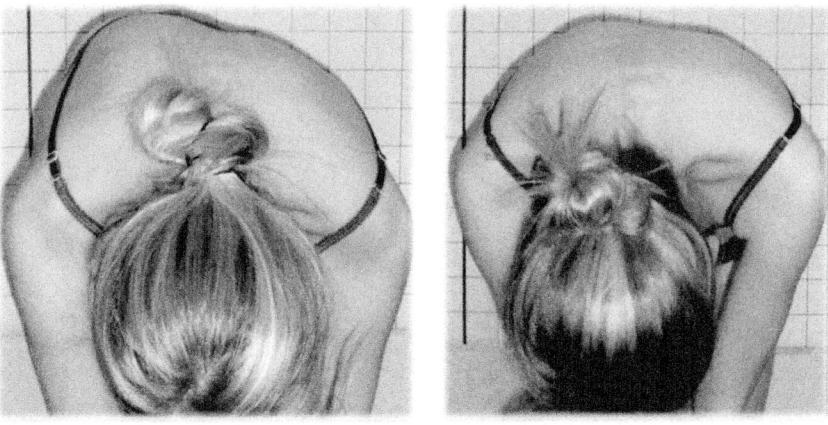

Fig. 5.10: Girl with a right thoracic curve of 42° treated in a CAD / CAM Chêneau brace of the Gensingen library with an intermediate correction of the rib hump as visible on the right.

Treatment teams with above-average end results have hitherto endeavored to use their braces to accomplish an optimum corrective effect on the X-ray, while at the same time training their patients in such a way that they can wear the brace all day during the growth spurt as much as possible. However, good radiological results do not always imply a favorable cosmetic outcome! Despite the fact that the curvature was clearly corrected on the X-ray at the conclusion of treatment, the rib hump often remained clearly visible; with some braces, there was even a cosmetically disturbing and extremely stiff case of flatback *(Fig. 5.11)*.

The X-ray only portrays the spine on one plane, while scoliosis is, properly speaking, a three-dimensional deformity with lateral curvature and distortion. Precisely because the X-ray has been in the forefront to such an extent up until now for assessing different treatment strategies, non-operative treatment has been capable of regularly contributing to the formation of flatback. The Boston brace is not the only brace to be known to regularly lead to flatback formation: German treatment concepts derived from wearing a Chêneau brace also once cause this functional disturbance, even though the curvature on the X-ray occasionally appears to be well corrected using such braces.

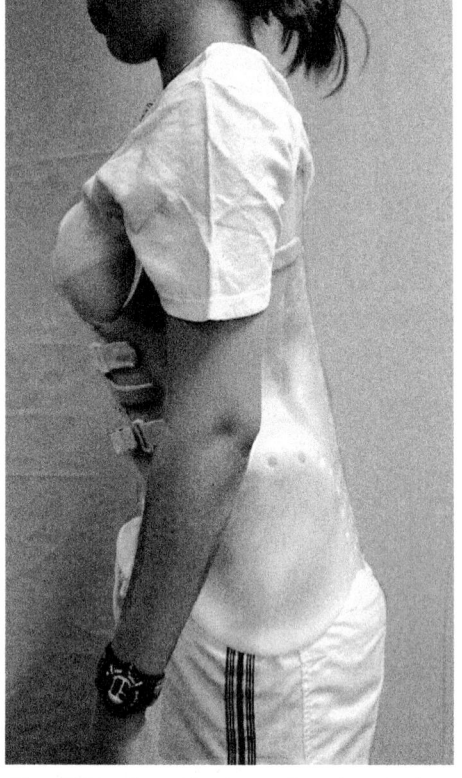

Fig. 5.11: Lateral view of a brace that promotes "flatback." The normal spinal curvatures are prevented by the brace. Stiffening occurs in an erect position.

Since the objective of brace treatment is not to straighten the image on the X-ray and send the patient home with a stiff case of flatback, the original Chêneau brace has been further developed in the 90s of the last century.

Still today we find braces without any correction of the sagittal profile (lateral view). These certainly cannot be seen as evidence based. Within the Gensingen Brace (GBW) approach the sagittal plane correction is constantly addressed *(Fig. 5.12)*.

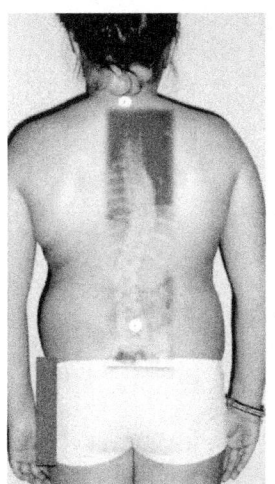 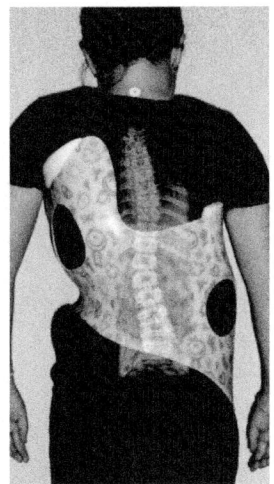 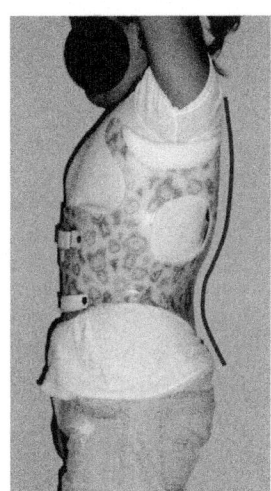

Fig. 5.12: A Gensingen brace produced in Greece on the recent standard. Besides the corrective movement in frontal plane (view from the *rear*) also a correction of the lateral view clearly is visible. Lumbar lordosis (hollowback) and thoracic kyphosis (roundback) both are restored in this brace as can be seen on the *right* (with kind permission by Nicos Tournavitis).

It has since been demonstrated that the best cosmetic results are obtained when, assuming a proper wearing time, there is a curvature correction of more than 20°, and additionally a distinct derotation as well. Seen from the side, the patients treated in this manner not only have a nearly normal spinal shape, but also practically normal spinal function. The stiff flatback caused by the outdated treatment concepts gives way to a functionally well-balanced spine with a good cosmetic result *(Figs. 5.13 a–d)*.

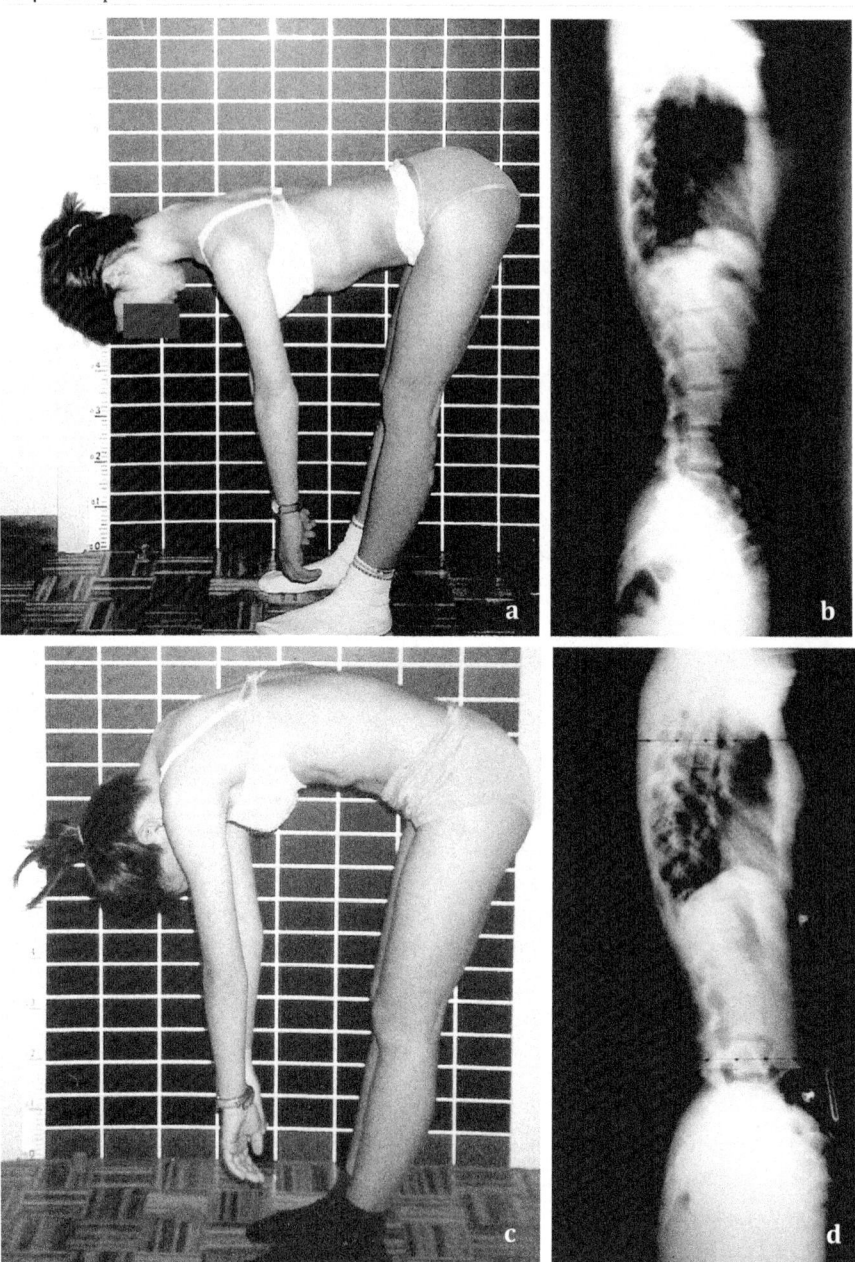

Figs. 5.13 a–d: Stiffened extreme flatback (a) also visible on the X-ray (b), caused by improper brace treatment. Below (c and d): After 12 months of treatment with a good Chêneau brace, practically normal conditions seen from the side (Weiss, Rigo, Chêneau 2000).

Chêneau himself pointed out at the beginning of the 1990s that scoliosis of the thoracic spine generally involves flatback and is to be treated accordingly with the brace. For this reason, good Chêneau braces are characterized by how they reproduce the sagittal curvature of the thoracic spine (lateral profile). This has also been consistently updated in the new plaster-free brace libraries, which are produced with computer assistance. In contrast, however, restoring the hollow-back (lumbar lordosis) reduced by scoliosis in the lumbar region is unfortunately still neglected on a regular basis by most of the Chêneau derivatives as well as by most other brace forms. This is still the case, despite the fact that we have known for about five years that restoring the lumbar lordosis, as the hollow-back is called in specialist terminology, can correct scoliosis.[21] These research results were confirmed once again only recently.

5.2.1 Design Variants of Trunk Orthoses in Scoliosis Therapy

Corrective trunk braces made from a plaster cast that are designed for scoliosis treatment vary significantly with regard to their quality and their effectiveness. For the most part, braces made according to a plaster cast bear the signature of the technician making them. He is often specialized in certain curvature patterns and thereby also capable of attaining outstanding corrective effects for these, while corrections for other curvature patterns may end up being below average. Braces made by means of computer-aided design (CAD) that employs extensive expert-based databases are ideal for use with all curvature patterns. Moreover, such an expert-supported quality assurance may mitigate possible sources of error.

Some very high-quality systems enabling top-level braces to be made without a plaster cast have been on the market for years now.

While today most brace variants partially or even completely neglect to restore physiological or natural lumbar lordosis, the Chêneau light® brace

---

[21] van Loon PJ, Kühbauch BA, Thunnissen FB: Forced lordosis on the thoracolumbar junction can correct coronal plane deformity in adolescents with double major curve pattern idiopathic scoliosis. *Spine.* 2008, Apr 1;33(7):797–801.

that is no longer available[22] as well as the Chêneau-Gensingen Brace® led to a marked correction of lumbar lordosis that is typically reduced in idiopathic scoliosis.

The Chêneau brace in its updated form and with the design variants that are now possible have solved the problems presented with other braces and has elevated brace making to a new level. The Boston brace as well as all other brace variants with an abdominal press end up aggravating flat back, which is precisely what has to be avoided as much as possible in light of the knowledge that the concomitant loss of hollow back favors chronic back pain in adults.

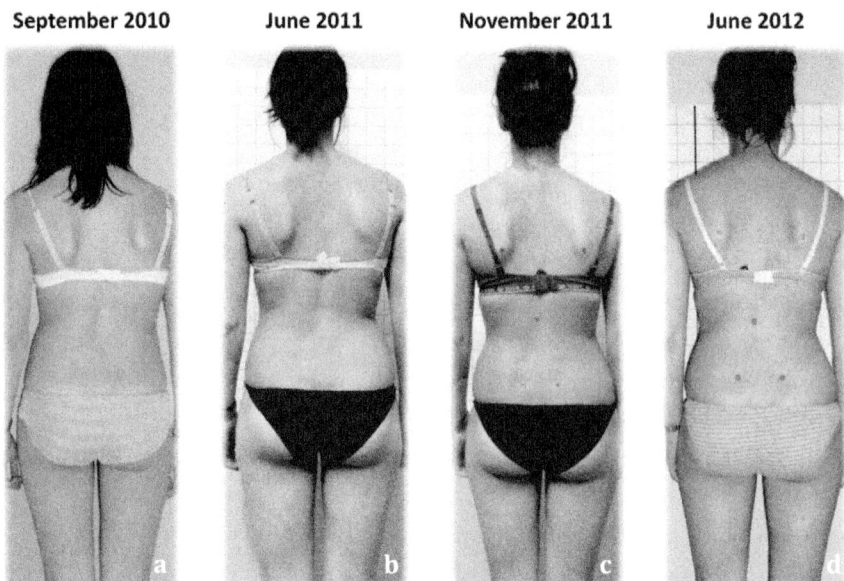

Figs. 5.14 a–d: A 13-year-old girl with a thoracic curvature of more than 50° at the beginning of treatment, treated with a Chêneau-Gensingen brace. At the end of treatment, there is good balance and a trunk symmetry that reveals almost no sign of scoliosis. (From: Weiss HR, Moramarco M. *Remodeling of trunk and backshape deformities in patients with scoliosis using standardized asymmetric CAD / CAM braces. Hard Tissue 2013 Feb 26;2(2):14.*)

---

[22] Weiss HR, Moramarco M. Remodelling of trunk and backshape deformities in patients with scoliosis using standardized asymmetric computer-aided design/computer-aided manufacturing braces. Hard Tissue 2013 Feb 26;2(2):14.

Meanwhile, it has been demonstrated that it is not only possible to ably correct even scoliosis with higher degree values by using modern Chêneau braces *(Fig. 5.14)*, but also that successful brace treatment can achieve cosmetic improvements in such cases that are comparable to those resulting from surgery.[13] However, brace treatment for higher-degree curvatures will only manage to be relatively pain-free if the necessary corrective measures with respect to the lateral profile, i.e. consistent correction of flat back, have been taken into account. In the meantime, there is considerable evidence pointing to the fact that the corrective effects of severely painful brace treatment regimens are not forfeited when a non-painful brace providing good lateral profile correction is used instead *(Figs. 5.15 a–f)*.

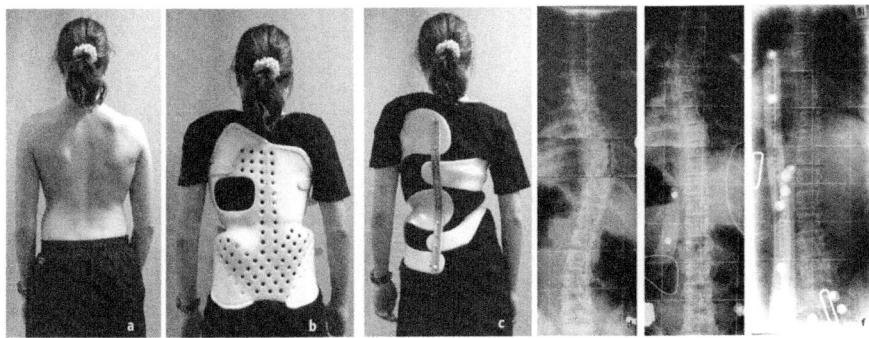

Figs. 5.15 a-f: A 13-year-old girl with thoracic-type adolescent idiopathic scoliosis of 39° according to Cobb. In the kyphoscoliotic brace, high thoracic 22°, thoracic 12°, lumbar 5°; in the Chêneau light brace high thoracic 22°, thoracic 8°, and lumbar 11°. In the lumbar area, the corrective force was purposely reduced in order to better compensate the appearance after brace treatment. There was severe pain with the brace in illustration (b), which disappeared after switching over to the brace in (c).

Corrective Effect in the Brace

The corrective effect in the brace, hitherto always given in % of the initial value, determines the final result within certain limits. But what is the use of an excellent X-ray if a stiffened flat back is incurred with functional loss and pain. Furthermore, the issue of stiffened curvatures leads to the following questions: Is it worthwhile wearing the brace if the corrective effect is slight? How can the percentage of the corrective effect be assessed for major curvatures?

In principle, the corrective effect is of great significance. According to Landauer,[23] at least 40% of primary correction is necessary for a sustained improvement (–7°). What should therefore be striven for is to constantly exceed this percentage correction, which will ensure that brace treatment is also worthwhile. Naturally, however, not all curvatures are equally correctable. It all depends on the curvature pattern, curvature strength, and individual stiffening. At 38°, we sometimes experience overcorrection to –14, and then – in contrast – a correction from 40° to just 38°, despite the fact that the braces designed according to the current state of knowledge using a standardized CAD system can necessarily be regarded as superior in quality *(Fig. 5.16)*.

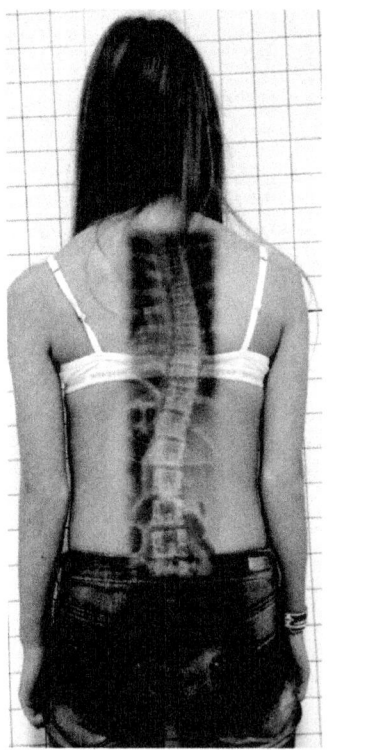 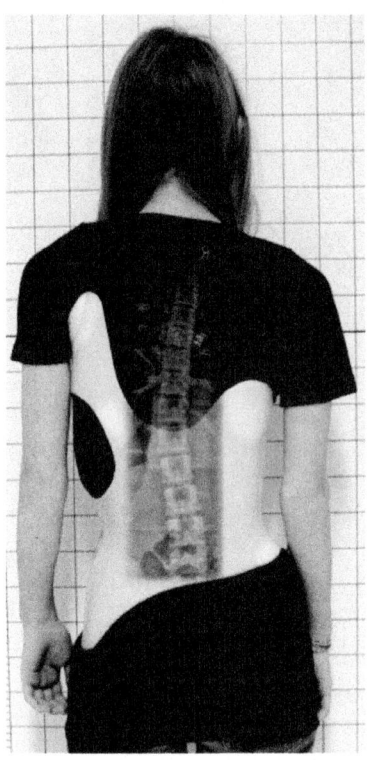

Figs. 5.16: Single curve patterns can be overcorrected when the curve is not too large and too stiff.

---

[23] Landauer F, Wimmer C, Behensky H. (2003) Estimating the final outcome of brace treatment for idiopathic thoracic scoliosis at 6-month follow-up. Pediatr Rehabil. 6(3–4):201–7.

The average corrective effect can, however, be markedly improved even for curvatures with more pronounced stiffening. Accordingly, a well-made and fitted brace is usually effective even when the corrective effect is slight, enabling curvature increase to at least be halted in most cases. Curvatures beyond the 60° limit can only be corrected by 50% in rare instances. Due to the fact that, with greater curvatures, even corrections of less than 40% have led to sustained curvature corrections in individual cases *(Figs. 5.17)*,[24] it is certainly worth considering whether the absolute correction attained, expressed in angular degrees, might not be better suited for establishing a prognosis than a percentage correction. In our experience, a corrective effect of at least 15° should be attained for curvatures beyond the 50° limit in order to stop progression. With 20° correction and above, we have accomplished permanent corrections even with curvatures exceeding 50°.

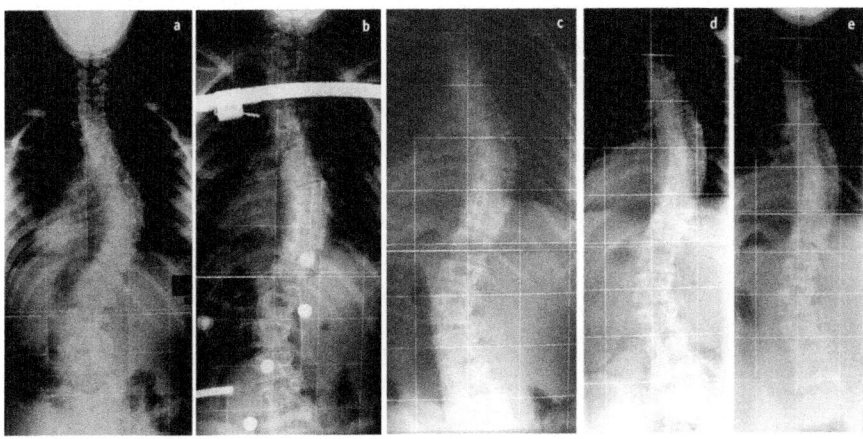

Figs. 5.17 a-e: A 13-year-old girl with thoracic progredient condition at 62° with qualitatively insufficient initial treatment in December 1995 (a). Correction in the new brace to 46° in January 1996 (b). 47°/40° (February 1998, c); 45°/40° (April 2001 after weaning off the brace, d); and 41°/37° (November 2002, 20 months after weaning off the brace, e). The condition is stable even in 2007, six years after weaning off the brace, and the patient has gone into business on her own as a hairdresser. She does not feel cosmetically impaired. Weiss HR (2007) Differentialindikation der Rumpforthesen in der Skoliosebehandlung, MOT 127.

---

[24] Weiß HR (2007) Differentialindikation der Rumpforthesen in der Skoliosebehandlung, MOT 127.

During brace treatment, the problems needing to be solved are not always covered by normal orthopedic or technical orthopedic training. Since scoliosis requiring treatment is a rarity anyway in orthopedic practice, conservative scoliosis management should only be done by treatment teams with appropriate experience, an adequate number of patients, and corresponding further training in this field.

Correction on the X-Ray / Cosmetic Correction

The corrective effect in the brace and the collaboration of those affected (compliance) are two decisive parameters for successful treatment. As long as we measure treatment effectiveness with the X-ray and use the Cobb angle as a parameter for determining success, we will only wind up with an inadequate view of the overall treatment results. While it is true that the Cobb angle is an important measurement parameter, it does not, however, reveal anything with respect to three-dimensional changes or cosmetic improvements.

As is known from the study of Appelgren and Willner (1990), many braces tend to aggravate the flat back typically associated with thoracic scoliosis, thus exposing patients to the risk of mechanical functional impairment that in certain circumstances may even lead to complaints.

In current brace variants made according to a precise pattern, the central concern – apart from correcting lateral deviation – is the restoration of the normal spinal curvature of the lateral profile. The starting point of the modeling technique is the idea that it needs to be possible to restore the kyphotic (outwardly round) components in the thoracic area and the lordotic (outwardly hollow) components in the lumbar region. This form must be given by the brace. Skilled pressure distribution that only permits kyphotic expansion of the thorax (back rounding) may be successful in restoring the lateral profile without bringing about other cosmetic defects in the thoracic region.

It has been demonstrated that it is possible for a good brace to reestablish kyphosis of the thoracic spine. When treating lumbar scoliosis, the restoration of lumbar lordosis needs to be incorporated in the same fashion, as it is typically reduced in such cases.

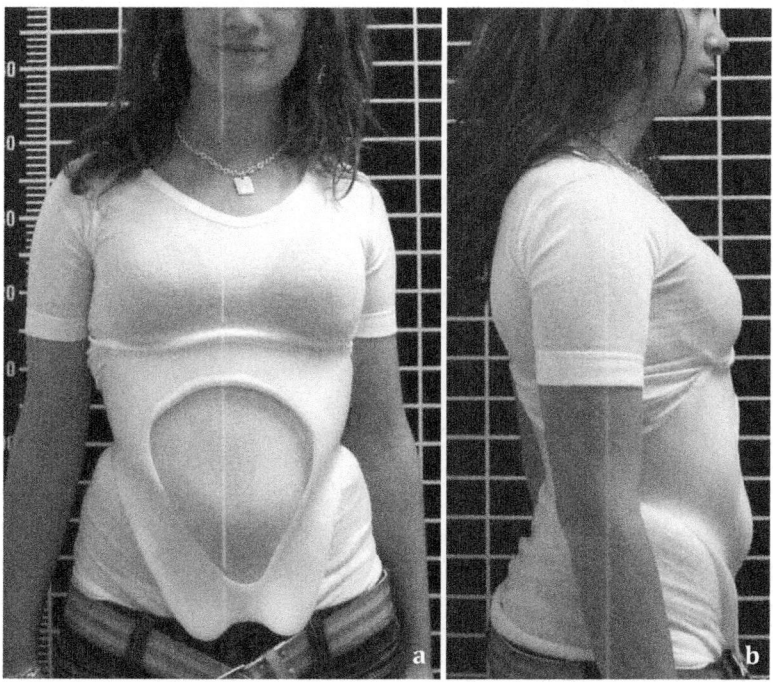

Figs. 5.18 a and b: So-called physio-logic® style brace seen from the front (a) and from the side (b).

According to the latest scientific findings, correcting the lateral profile flattened in scoliosis also has a positive effect on lateral deviation and on spinal rotation. This treatment principle has materialized in the so-called physio-logic® brace, which is able to correct scoliosis of the lumbar spine *(Figs. 5.18 a and b)*. This brace can be used when "normal" brace treatment is not possible due to a concomitant disease or a lack of collaboration on the part of the patient. Long-term results for patients during the main growth spurt are not yet available, which is why this brace is only to be recommended when the above-mentioned restriction applies. However, this brace has already proven itself in the medium term in adult scoliosis patients with complaints of pain *(Figs. 5.19 a and b)*. Prior to its use, the effect of the brace can be simulated by a motion test to find out whether this treatment principle has the potential to be effective for the case being examined.[25]

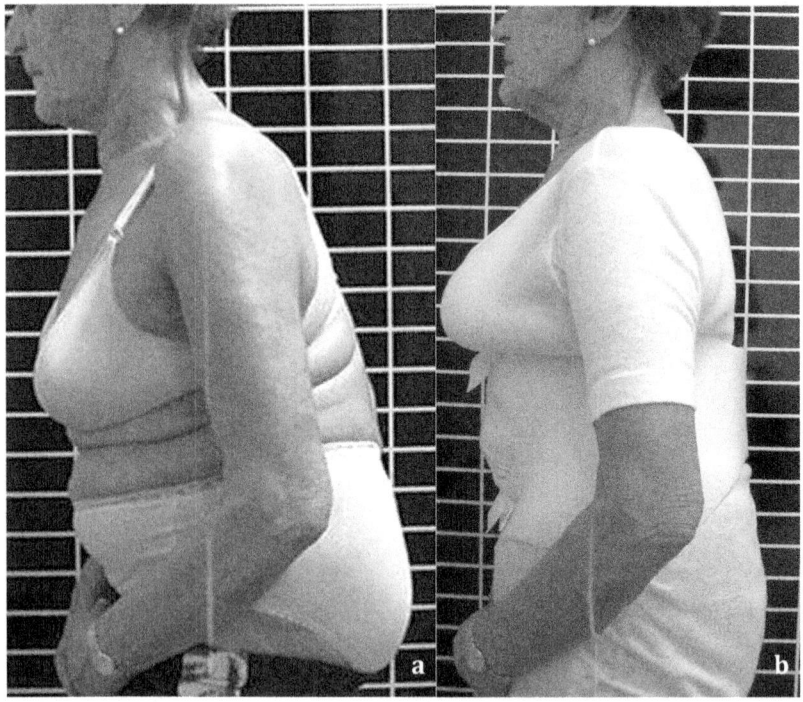

Figs. 5.19 a and b: First generation physio-logic® brace used here to treat pain in a female patient with severe thoracolumbar scoliosis and chronic low-back pain. The straightening effect is very visible.

Psychological Problems Related to Brace Treatment

Wearing a brace during the main growth spurt for 23 hours a day considerably decreases the quality of life, which is why very few patients are actually enthusiastic about wearing their brace. If qualitatively different consultations leave the afflicted feeling insecure, it is not surprising that they ultimately refuse the essential factor of participating in their treatment. The girls being treated are frequently ashamed to show their braces, and so their

---

[25] Weiss HR: Das "Sagittal Realignment Brace" (physio-logic® brace) in der Behandlung von erwachsenen Skoliosepatienten mit chronifiziertem Rückenschmerz (MOT 2005; 125: 45–54).

wearing time unfortunately amounts to a maximum of 16 hours, which is insufficient during the main growth spurt to gain improvements.

However, understanding and empathy usually help to improve the wearing time, especially if the parents manage to get their own feelings under control and deal with the issues more calmly. The situation frequently proves very unsettling for parents. What is more, they often feel guilty ("How could this have happened at all?") and are now looking for the "best way" for their children "as fast as possible." They make inquiries all over the place, including via the Internet, which leads to even greater uncertainty thanks to "self-appointed" amateurs – usually afflicted themselves – who believe they have found a meaningful and successful field in their newly acquired role. Unfortunately, this sometimes results in a good brace being replaced by a new one and good advice losing out to an unprofessional "second opinion."

The mental stress that children and their parents are subjected to when making decisions can hardly be dealt with without psychological support. Only in very few cases are the fears and self-reproach justified; such feelings are by no means a good basis for arriving at decisions, and they all too often prevent the best possible treatment from being successful.

It is clear that brace treatment compromises the quality of life of those affected, which is why it is not only important for specialists to incorporate the latest technical advances in their work, but also for them to further develop brace treatment until it is an *established fact* that the impairment of the quality of life is offset by successful treatment, a treatment that reliably averts operations and, what is more, leaves every treated patient satisfied as well.

5.2.2 Learning to Wear a Brace

Once the trial fitting and initial changes for improving the wearing comfort of the brace have been carried out, it should immediately be worn as constantly as possible throughout the main growth spurt. To relieve pressure, it is sufficient in most cases to simply open the clasps of the brace for 15–20 minutes and then re-tighten them. These periods of rest allow the skin to recover, thus enabling the body to frequently tolerate an uninterrupted wearing time of more than 20 hours even on the first day. Generally, after it has been worn for about a week, the brace will then be tolerated for 23 hours straight. However, if there is any difficulty sleeping while learning to wear the brace full-time, I recommend waiting 3 days before trying to wear the brace at night again. Otherwise, the loss of sleep from the repeated attempts to wear the brace night after night can have a demoralizing effect.

When getting used to wearing the brace, any complaints should be taken seriously, meaning that it is extremely important to recognize and eliminate problem areas, so that at the end of the wearing-in period of the brace, the only pressure still felt is at the necessary pressure points.

If the truss pad covers a large patch of skin around the main pressure areas, then a good corrective effect will be achieved with a minimum amount of physical impairment. Pain occurs if there is no clearance (voids) in the brace for the pressure areas. The lack of such clearance squeezes the trunk, which is not generally tolerated. The solution to this problem does not come from reducing the pressure (and thus impoverishing the corrective effect), but by taking care of the lack of clearance areas! Unfortunately, the clearance areas make the brace a little bulkier, but this is precisely the way to achieve the best effect. Should there still be pain even after all of the brace's deficiencies have been eliminated, it will be necessary for the patient to be re-examined in detail. In individual cases, rib blocking may prevent the brace from being tolerated. In such instances, physiotherapy, manual therapy, or even chirotherapy should be tried to get rid of the pain caused by functional issues; medications and massages, medicinal baths, electrotherapy, or simply rest may also be prescribed if there is costovertebral joint inflammation.

Another part of the process of getting used to wearing the brace is being given extensive information and answers to every question. Patients often come to the consultation sessions with their parents. If in the course of the conversation and examination it becomes evident that the parents tend to react emotionally, it is advisable for the attending doctor to first talk with them alone and present the issues in a disarming manner. In many cases, emotionally charged remarks made by the parents lead to the child declining the necessary brace treatment or viewing it as something awful. At the same time, the attending physician should not overplay his hand, but rather allow the child or adolescent to be responsible for making the decision on his or her own as much as possible. Showing understanding and providing ample information is usually more than sufficient to awaken a sense of personal responsibility even in children under 10 years of age, thus contributing to a favorable course of treatment. Sometimes, parents who are overzealous must even be held back from admonishing their child multiple times a day, particularly as warnings in this phase of personality development might foster resistance and result in the brace being refused. It is therefore better for the child to successfully get used to wearing the brace 14 days later than for the brace to be rejected outright.

At the start of the wearing-in phase of the brace, it is sometimes necessary to treat the pressure points of the skin by brushing them and rubbing in alcohol. Creams should generally be avoided, as they soften the skin, thereby making it less resistant to pressure.

However, the latest developments – such as the Chêneau-Gensingen brace – are already standardized and fine-tuned to such an extent that the above-described skin care only needs to be recommended when treating curvatures beyond the 60° limit. This is because hardly any more skin irritations occur within the normal range of indications. A slight reddening of the skin is, however, normal at the beginning of brace treatment.

5.2.3 Treatment Duration and Weaning off the Brace

Treatment duration can vary widely. Should the wearing-in period of the brace result in completely correcting or even overcorrecting a relatively slight curvature angle, it may well be that the process of weaning off the brace can be started after the onset of menstruation – before a marked curvature in the opposite direction ensues. In contrast, for more pronounced scoliosis curvatures (> 40°) that cannot be completely corrected it is necessary to wear the brace as long as possible. It used to be the case that girls almost always had their braces weaned off at the age of 15 or 16. It has been demonstrated, however, that longer wearing times lead to better (cosmetic) results. This can probably be attributed to the fact that spinal growth still partly continues for more than 2 years after the growth plates visible on the X-ray have closed. With more pronounced curvatures, therefore, while we begin weaning off the brace at age 16, we do not end this process until between the ages of 18 and 20, depending on the state of maturity.

The brace worn full time can be taken off for school sports. However, it has to be put back on again immediately afterwards in order for the wearing time not to be reduced unnecessarily. Competitive sports are mainly to be avoided by scoliosis patients with a brace if it could cause the spine to become hypermobile, which, however, does not rule out deciding in favor of competitive sports in individual cases (e.g. swimming).

In school sports, scoliosis patients are frequently disadvantaged. This is especially true for children and adolescents who wear a brace. In accordance with a resolution of the German Conference of Federal Ministers of Education and the Arts in 1988, diligence and commitment during physical education can be used in such cases as the basis for the grading assessment instead of performance. Unfortunately, this is implemented only very rarely – probably due to sheer ignorance – when a comparative assessment of physical education performance is not possible for medical reasons.

Should any problems surface when wearing a brace, such as pain, tingling sensations, or even nausea and shortness of breath, the attending orthopedist should be consulted. He will then carry out an exam to determine what the complaints can be attributed to. With technical problems with the brace (torn off clasp, cracked frame, etc.), the orthopedic technician should be directly addressed.

The X-rays necessary for the checkup result in a certain amount of radiation exposure. In slender persons, this can be reduced by taking checkup X-rays with the brace still on and with half the exposure time, therefore involving half as much radiation. The quality of the X-rays is still adequate for measuring the angle of curvature, even in very thin children, if all the details of the bone structure are recognizable *(Figs. 5.20)*. Even an overlay of the radiation field on the curvature area allows the radiation exposure to be reduced considerably.[26]

---

[26] Weiss HR, Seibel S (2013) Region of Interest (ROI) in the radiological follow-up of patients with scoliosis. Hard Tissue, June 1; 2(4):33

For the trunk muscles to be able to grow accustomed to being without the brace, it is necessary for them to be gradually weaned from wearing the brace at the conclusion of treatment. To do this, the wearing time is reduced by 3-4 hours a day to begin with for a period of 3 months, after which the brace is only worn at night for the last six months.

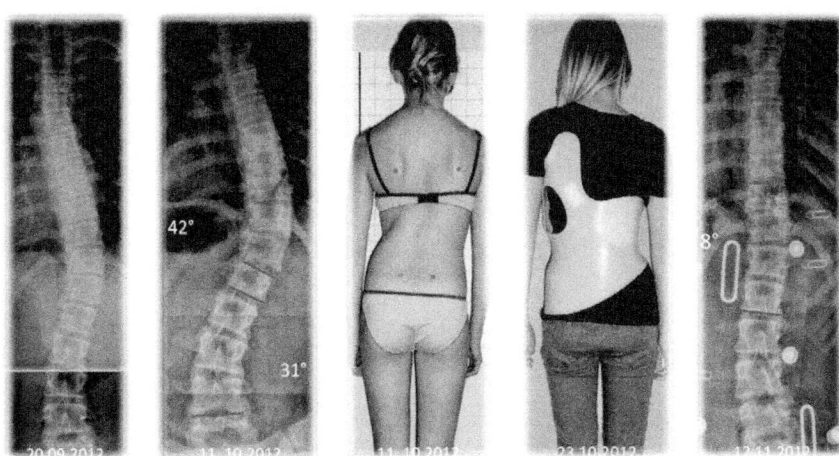

Fig. 5.20: Patient with scoliosis and vast progression in the short-term prior to brace treatment with the x-rays made according to the least possible exposure to radiation. The region of interest (ROI) is clearly visible and in this girl even with a reduction of the exposure time the structural entities of the bony tissue is visible.

5.2.4 Frequently Asked Questions (FAQ) – What Can Patients Expect from Bracing?

Brace treatment for patients with scoliosis can be regarded as a long-lasting impairment of the quality of life and therefore a great challenge. To undertake this task of brace treatment, the patient needs to be informed not only about the realistic aims of treatment, but also about problems arising from the spinal deformity itself. It is only under this precondition that the patient can decide for himself about brace treatment and also take responsibility for treatment.

The objective of this chapter is to address the most important issues involved with brace treatment. On the one hand addressing these issues of brace treatment seems beneficial for the professionals who regularly treat patients with scoliosis and, on the other hand, also appears to be necessary as there are so many inappropriate and scientifically unacceptable claims and statements currently made in the Internet media.

We have to minimize the fears of the patients and their families when, for example, people say, "A good brace has to be painful!" This is categorically untrue and yet it is found in many publications on the Internet.

Also, questions concerning the percentage of in-brace correction cannot be reduced to a simple number. Doing so causes uncertainty in patients and their parents, although there will sometimes be a beneficial outcome even with an in-brace correction of less than 50%. However, a true professional will not be satisfied with an in-brace correction of 50% when the curvature will easily permit a far greater amount of correction.

Therefore, it seems reasonable to differentiate in this matter and keep patients and their parents on the straight and narrow path to success.

The best possible in-brace correction is not worth a thing if the brace cannot be worn!

The following is a brief list of questions that arise on a daily basis in the practice of a conservative scoliosis specialist and the appropriate answers based on scientific evidence.

1. Is brace treatment painful?

A good brace corrects the deformity to the best possible extent without leading to pain. An actual correction can only take place when there is room for the corrective movement, not by applying compressive forces.

Sometimes the corrective effect of compression braces can be very satisfactory, but this correction is pointless if the brace cannot be worn due to pain. An unpublished study from Stuttgart (Germany) investigating the use of compression braces by a special sample of scoliosis patients showed excellent in-brace corrections; however, 50% of the patients dropped out of the study because they were not able to wear their brace, thus making this study worthless.

2. Is an in-brace correction greater than 50% always achievable with braces of the highest possible standard?

Since the in-brace correction is dependent on a variety of factors, this question clearly must be answered with: **No!**

There are patient-dependent factors:
- Curve pattern
- Patient age
- Curvature stiffness
- Capability of the patient
- Compliance

Brace-dependent factors are:
- Pattern specificity
- Shifting of the trunk areas against each other
- Exact fitting

Double (triple) curve patterns allow far less correction than single curve patterns. The curve of an 11-year-old girl can be corrected more easily than the curve of a 16-year-old girl with comparable Cobb angles and comparable curve patterns wearing the same brace model.

According to recent scientific knowledge the in-brace correction should exceed 15°; however, in stiff curvatures this does not always seem possible *(see Figs. 5.21–5.24)*. Nevertheless, a professional will not readily accept a low in-brace correction, and when the pattern of curvature in the brace is obviously not reflected, the lack of in-brace correction cannot be explained by curvature stiffness. It is only when a brace is designed according to the current "state-of-the-art" standard and when improvements to the adjustment do not lead to an increased in-brace correction that the lack of correction can be attributed to the stiffness of the curvature. However, only the experienced specialist will be able to distinguish between these facts.

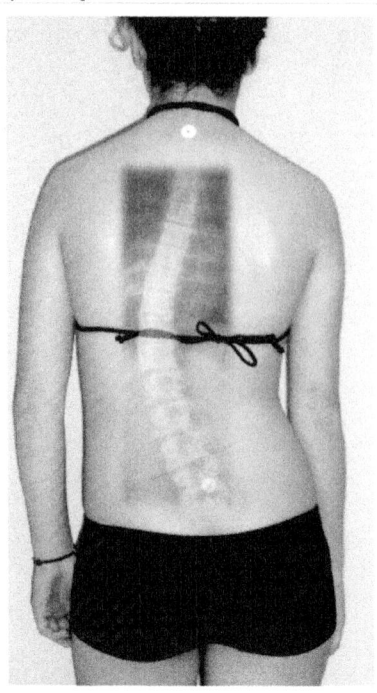
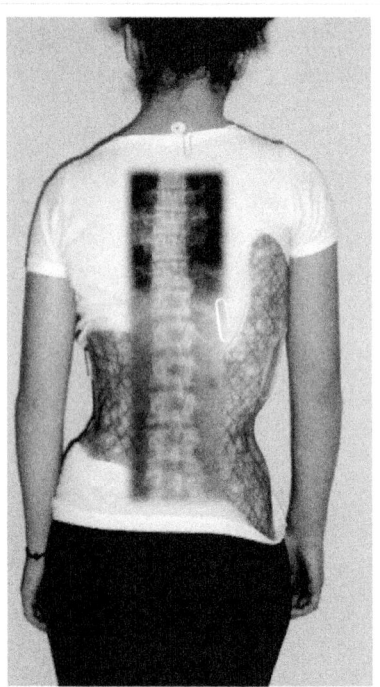

Fig. 5.21: Full correction in a single thoracic curve pattern (with kind permission by Nicos Tournavitis).

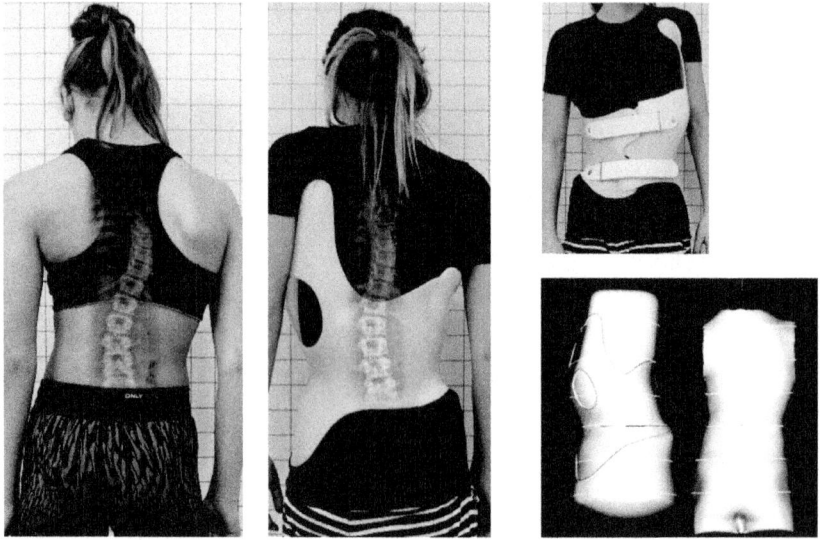

Fig. 5.22: More than 50% of correction in a girl with a thoracic curve exceeding 45° in a GBW. On the *right* the patients scan and the patients CAD brace is visible.

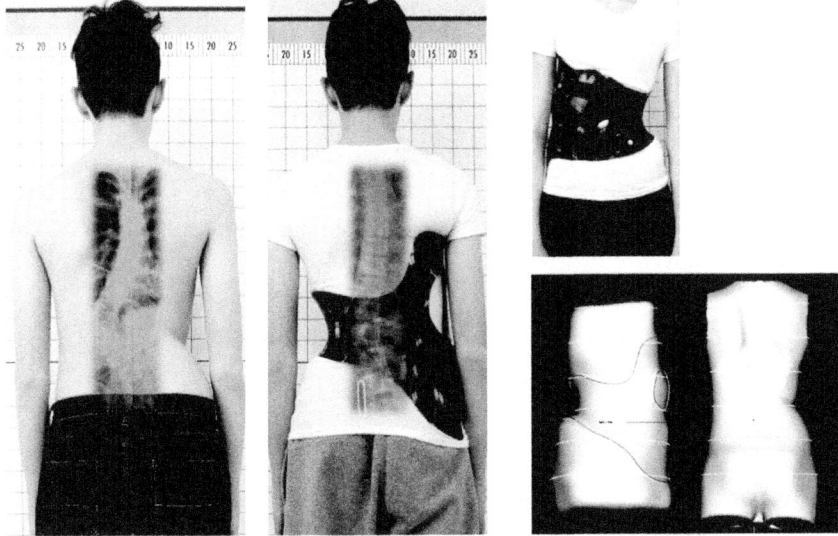

Fig. 5.23: More than 50% of correction in a boy with a thoracolumbar curve exceeding 60° in a GBW. On the *right* the patients scan and the patients CAD brace is visible.

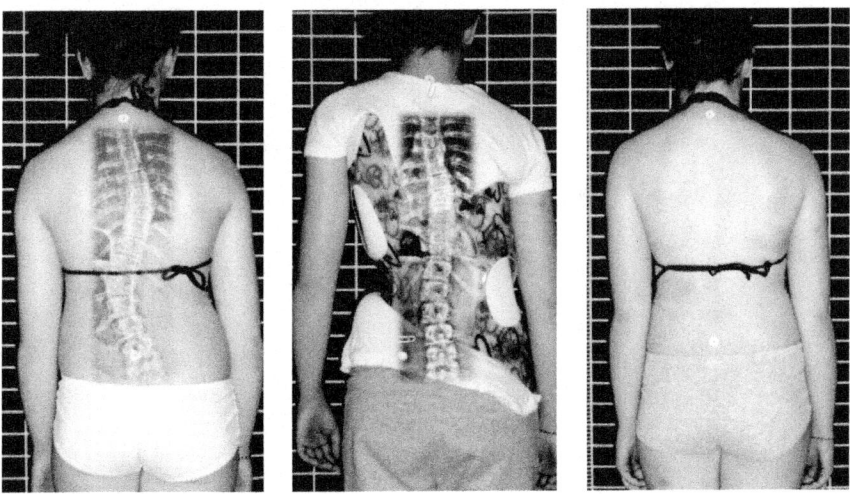

Fig. 5.24: More than 50% of correction in a girl with a double curve pattern. After 6 weeks of brace treatment a slight clinical correction already is visible (*right*).

3. Do I need to be braced with a curvature of 20°?

This question can only be addressed when a wider range of facts and information are taken into account. A 7-year-old child usually has not yet reached the pubertal growth spurt *(Fig. 5.25)* and, therefore, does not yet need a brace, or only requires nighttime bracing. A 16-year old girl with 20° curvature usually has no further residual growth and does not need any more treatment.

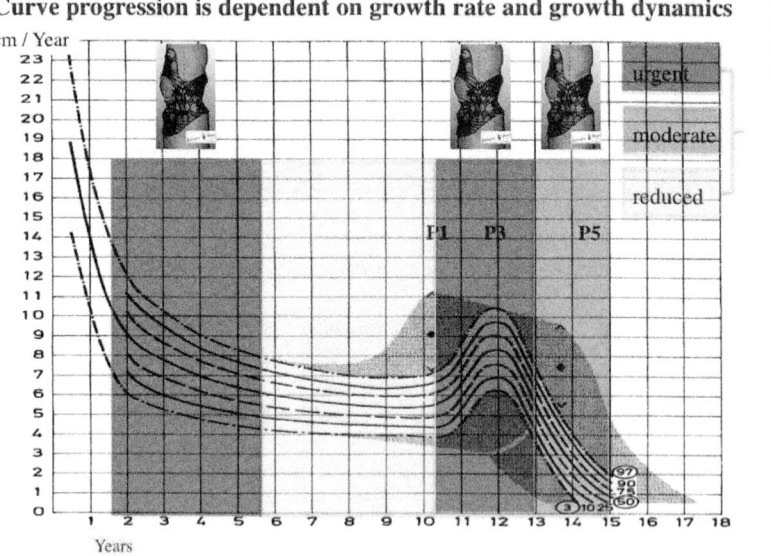

Growthrate (body length) as estimated for girls

Modified acc. to: Simon C: Klinische Pädiatrie, Schattauer

Fig. 5.25: The growth curve for girls: Between age 6 and the onset of the first signs of maturity, there is generally no significant increase in curvature that occurs. Once the first signs of maturity ensue (P1), a considerable increase in curvature can be expected. Depending on the severity of the curvature, therefore, timely brace treatment may be necessary, since an increase in curvature can occur within only a few weeks during the main growth spurt.

However, an 11-year-old girl with 20°, according to current knowledge, needs full-time bracing because she is in the pubertal growth spurt, at >80% risk for being progressive and can usually be corrected easily.

If a patient is braced at an early stage when a good in-brace correction can be achieved, there is a real chance for the brace wearing time to be reduced if the curve is below 15° after 6 months of brace treatment. This is not as easy in more mature patients with larger angles of curvature.

During the pubertal growth spurt curvatures of 15° should also be braced at least part-time, especially when there is a large deformity in comparison to the Cobb angle (large rotation, slight lateral deviation). In such a case if no treatment is undertaken a bad prognosis can be assumed, as well as a reduction of "participation" due to the deformity of the trunk.

4. What can be regarded as successful brace treatment?

When a curve with a high risk of being progressive is kept stable within the limits of the accepted measuring error (+/- 5°) until growth ends, this can be regarded as successful brace treatment. For the Boston brace the success rate seems to be 70%, and for the old Chêneau brace (Standard 1999) 80%. According to recent publications the success rate of the CAD / CAM Chêneau brace (Gensingen library) is over 90% and in curvatures between 20 and 40° a final correction of the curve and deformity can be achieved when the brace is worn full-time during residual growth *(Fig. 5.26-5.28.)*.

Nevertheless, even in patients of relative maturity and with little residual growth remaining, cosmetic improvements (e.g. a recomposition of the trunk) can be achieved using braces of the latest standard. Such cosmetic improvements significantly reduce deformity-dependent stress that the patient might experience and thereby reduce the desire to undergo surgery.

Unfortunately, even patients being treated with the best possible brace may quit. Growth dynamics cannot be predicted and sometimes the brace—initially adjusted properly—is very unsuitable at a checkup due to patient growth. When it is decided at the checkup to leave the brace as it is or with minor corrections for another 3 months and the patient grows drastically at this stage, the curvature can even increase in rare cases because of the fast growth and unpredictable growth timing (growth peak at the wrong time). This makes the brace no longer suitable; yet braces cannot be renewed too often due to the cost that this would incur.

Finally, a significant end-result correction, as seen on the X-ray, can only be achieved in patients with much residual growth and full brace-wearing time. In more mature individuals (girls 14, boys 16 years of age) residual progression can easily be stopped and an improvement to the clinical aspect (cosmesis) is possible. However, as in improvements after surgery, there is no proof to date that the improvements achieved with a brace can be regarded as stable in the long-term.

In curvatures beyond 40° significant and stable improvements persisting 5 years after brace weaning seem to be rare; however, progression can be stopped in most of these cases using recent CAD/CAM-based Chêneau derivates *(Fig. 5.29)*.

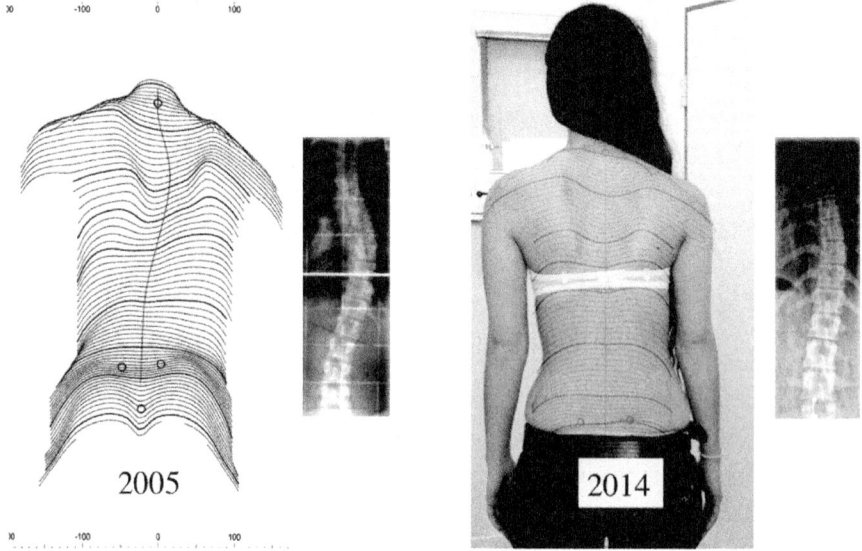

Fig. 5.26: Girl with a 38° thoracic curvature at the start of treatment with a significant deformity as visible in the surface scan *(left)*. On the *right* long term result 5.6 years after brace weaning 19° showing that corrections achieved with braces of the recent generation may be stable in the long-term.

5.2 Brace Treatment | 97

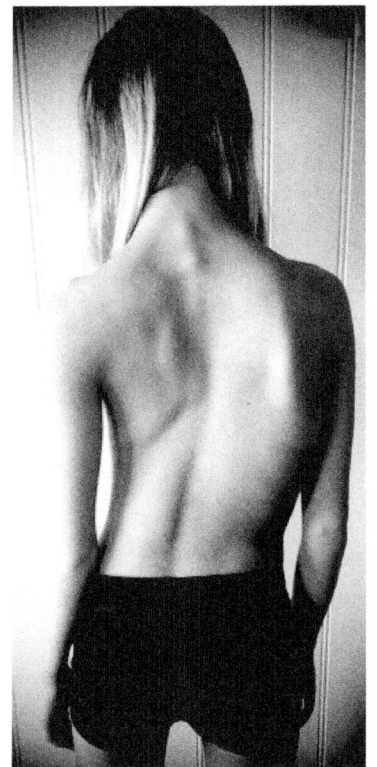 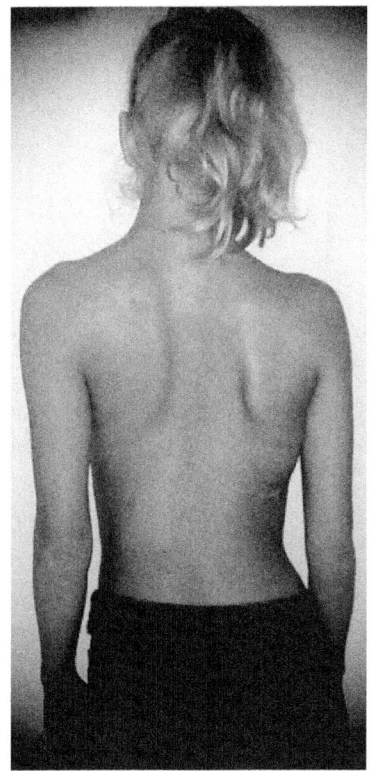

Fig. 5.27: Clinical improvement after only six weeks of wearing time.

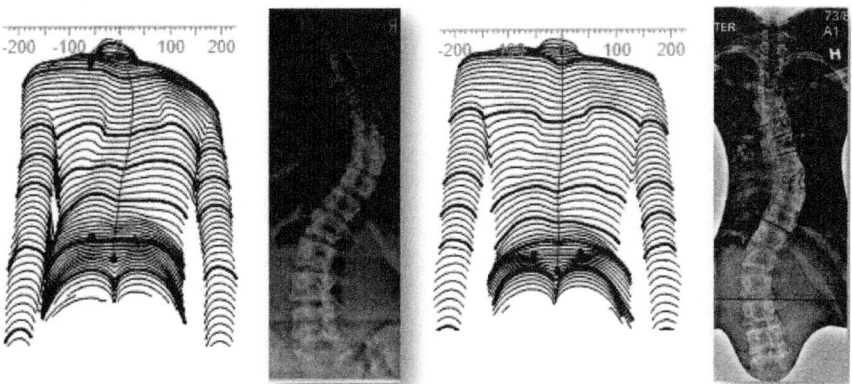

Fig. 5.28: Cosmetic and radiologic intermediate result after 4 months of wearing a Gensingen Brace (GBW).

98 | Chapter 5. Treatment

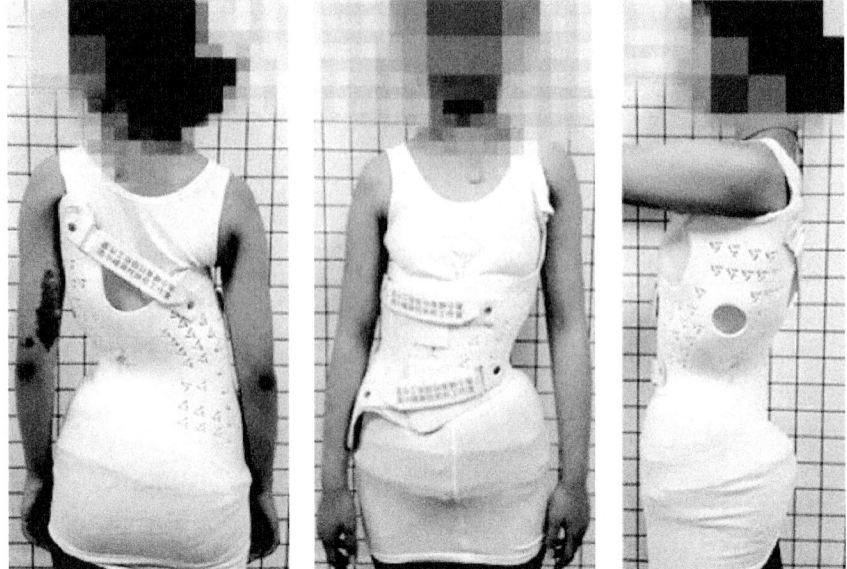

Fig. 5.29: Recent technology: Gensingen brace printed in 3D in China (Xiaofeng Nan). This brace for a double major curve enabled to correct both curves in full.

5. How long will it be necessary to wear the brace?

The main indication for brace treatment as a growth channelling treatment is during the different phases of growth. During the main growth phase a progression of 20 to 40° may occur within a few weeks in an unbraced patient. At the end of the pubertal growth phase (15 years of age in girls and 17 years in boys), there will usually be no progression exceeding 15° within a single year. We should, however, bear in mind the fact that even at the end of the pubertal growth spurt significant improvements to balance and clinical appearance are possible when the treatment is performed with a "Best Practice" brace, and therefore brace treatment may also be important during this time to improve patient collaboration and reduce the patient's desire to undergo surgery.

When an overcorrection in immature patients can be gained *(Fig. 5.30)* the parents should be advised to check their children every two weeks and have a presentation in the professionals office every 6 weeks.

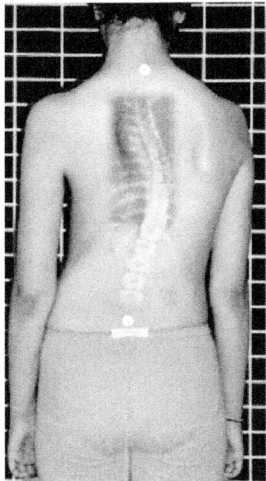 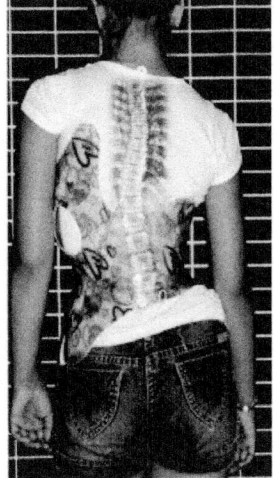 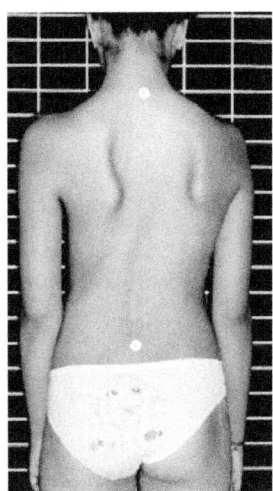

Fig. 5.30: Overcorrection in a thoracic curve with a significant Cobb angle and with some cosmetic improvement within the first 6 weeks under treatment with a Gensingen Brace (GBW). In such immature patients the parents should be advised to check their children every two weeks and have a presentation in the professionals office every 6 weeks! With kind permission from SBPRS, Thessaloniki (Nicos Tournavitis).

When clinical overcorrection has been reached brace wearing time must be reduced from > 20 hours to 16 hours per day. If there still is overcorrection we reduce to 12 hours. If the clinical correction then is reduced again we go back to more hours and finally with this kind of management we can produce the best possible clinical outcome and the best possible balance of the trunk. In many cases we can reduce the brace wearing time already at a time when the patient is still immature.

In a compliant patient with a curvature of less than 30° at the initiation of treatment, weaning can be started at the age of 15 years in girls and 17 years in boys. In curvatures exceeding 30° at the start of treatment, brace weaning should be started later and should last longer in order to allow for stabilization of the results achieved.

Naturally the curvature increases to some extent after brace weaning is completed. This should not be regarded as deterioration. Even when waiting one year longer for weaning in a patient with an initial curvature of less than 30°, the curvature would increase to the same extent.

6. Is it necessary to undergo physiotherapy continuously during brace treatment?

Brace treatment is absolutely essential during a pubertal growth spurt (see also Fig. 7.2) and curve pattern specific exercise instruction based on Schroth principles can provide an added advantage if the patient can tolerate both the brace and an exercise program. The importance of learning how to avoid postures that will increase the curvature and overload the spine during daily activities when the patient is out of the brace cannot be underestimated. Intensive treatment of three to five sessions of 90 minutes, twice per day, should be sufficient to achieve this goal.

Physiotherapy performed in specialized and certified centres can offer added value in terms of psychological support to the patient during brace treatment. However, if physiotherapy is perceived as being stressful and overly burdensome for the patient, it seems reasonable for him or her to go on with brace treatment alone during the pubertal growth spurt.

If the patient does forgoe therapy during bracing, it is advisable at the time of weaning to start a short program of rehabilitation in order for the patient to learn to avoid harmful postures which could negatively affect the benefits derived from bracing.

5.2.5 Future Developments in Brace Treatment – a Perspective

With the advent of CAD technology, it has become possible to further reinforce the corrections right up to the limit of what is tolerable *(Fig. 5.29)*. Yet more pronounced trunk displacement would, in turn, be very conspicuous in everyday life and keep the persons affected from wearing such a "lopsided" brace at school.

Possible future prospects might be a combined application, such as by carrying out maximum-correction treatment not tolerable in everyday life for 8 to 12 hours in conjunction with a "biofeedback system," in other words a flexible correction device for daytime use that is no longer obvious at school and in leisure time. Unfortunately, the systems (soft braces) like these that have been introduced on the market so far are not suitable for a wide variety of reasons.

This is why the author has begun developing a new "biofeedback system" based on the most recent levels of scientific knowledge.

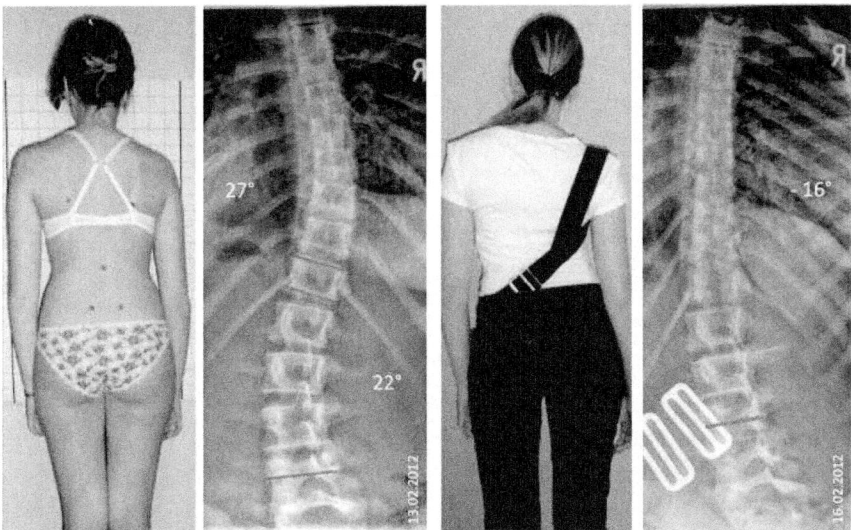

Fig. 5.31: A 12-year-old girl with a curvature of 28° according to Cobb that is still relatively flexible. In the Spinealite® biofeedback system, an overcorrection is evidence of the corrective potential, which, however, cannot be fully taken advantage of for adult-age patients.

This is relatively simple to apply. It cannot be considered as comfortable, however, since the correction occurs through traction on a shoulder. Wearing comfort also changes subject to the traction force set (correction). For adolescents, the maximum correction possible should be set, which entails sacrifices in comfort.

In adults with severe curvatures, however, we have had good experience with a milder correction traction.

Here, it is not a question of maximum correction, but rather preventing the trunk from drifting off to the side, which, by increasing in the course of the day, can tire the patient more and more and lead to complaints.

The corrective effect of this system was already able to be demonstrated *(Fig. 5.31)*; long-term results, however, are not yet available.

5.3 Operation and Surgical Procedures

If, despite all efforts, curvature continues to increase and the extent of curvature exceeds 50 degrees according to Cobb, an operation is generally recommended (German Guideline *"Idiopathic Scoliosis in Adolescence"*: http://www.awmf.org/leitlinien/detail/ll/033-025.html). To begin with, this begs the question: "Why an operation at all?"

In late onset, so-called adolescent idiopathic scoliosis, an operation is not necessarily required from a medical viewpoint, and to date there is no scientific evidence in support of the hypothesis that the resulting health conditions of scoliosis left as is would be considered as being worse than those following a scoliosis operation. It has been demonstrated that such curvatures do not, as a rule, grow so large that life-threatening restrictions on the cardiovascular system are to be feared. There is no correlation between scoliosis and pain either. For these patients, therefore, there needs to be another reason why they would decide to have themselves operated on with a curvature angle exceeding 50 degrees.

If the patient can avoid perceiving scoliosis as a curvature of his or her own spine or viewing it day by day as a "deformation," thereby suffering mental anguish and feeling depressed, out of sorts, and disadvantaged with respect to quality of life, then it is possible to do something about it. For then it is not the purely medical reasons, but the psychological viewpoints that determine the outlook. If there is no motivation for physiotherapy and brace treatment either, then no other therapeutical procedure is left for treating the deformity besides an operation.

According to the findings of health psychology, mental stress caused by the deformity may also lead to physical complaints.

Without a doubt, therefore, in such cases it is not a question of just a cosmetic operation. By no means should indications for surgery only depend on radiological findings if corresponding psychosocial impairments are not present *(Figs. 5.32 a–c)*!

With early onset curvatures and in some cases of congenital spinal scoliosis, which even in early infancy may be quite pronounced, an operation is justified very early on even for purely medical reasons. This sometimes applies to a subset of children with nerve and muscle disorders, as well as the often severe spinal deformities resulting from these underlying conditions. A Cochrane review, however, has not found evidence for spinal fusion surgery in neuromuscular scoliosis due to Duchenne muscular dystrophy.[27]

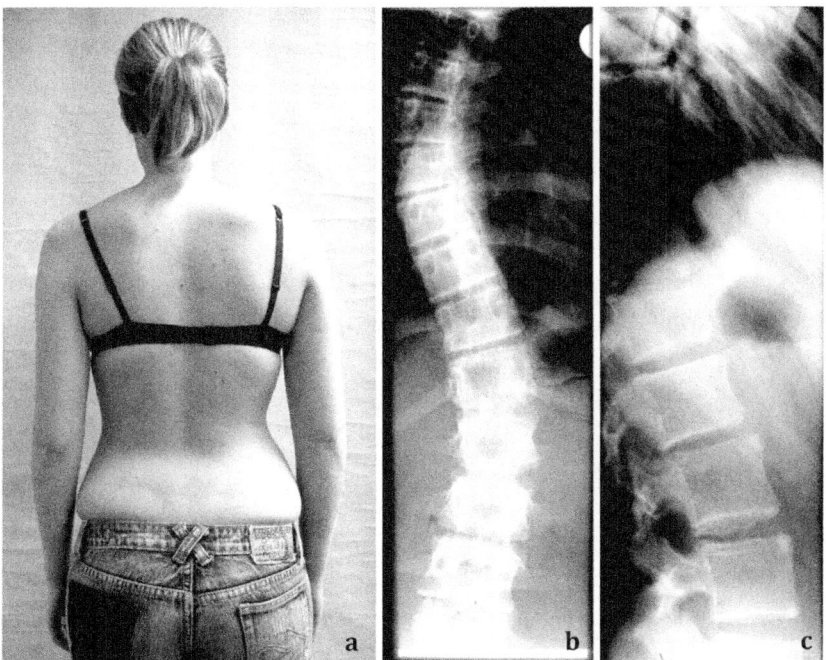

Figs. 5.32 a–c A 14-year-old patient, bone age 14.9, 98.8% mature, without any significant cosmetic impairment, satisfied with her appearance. Curvature angle: high thoracic 43°, low thoracic 32°. An urgent indication for surgery was determined! *Prognosis:* Only slight tendency towards progression, even without therapy; *no significant cosmetic deterioration to be expected!*

---

[27] Daniel KL Cheuk, Virginia Wong, Elizabeth Wraige, Peter Baxter, Ashley Cole. Surgery for scoliosis in Duchenne muscular dystrophy. Editorial Group: Cochrane Neuromuscular Disease Group. Published Online: 28 FEB 2013. Assessed as up-to-date: 31 JUL 2012.

What Surgical Procedures Are There?

Basically, we differentiate between posterior and anterior surgical access.

5.3.1 Posterior Access

With posterior access, the scars lie in the central line of the trunk, and it is usually necessary for there to be a scar above one of the two iliac crests. Various rod systems are currently being used for this operation. They are attached to the spine by hooks or – nowadays almost exclusively – by screws, thus spanning large sections. For better stabilization, these long rods are made with various cross connections to prevent any mobility at all in the spanned spinal region directly after the operation. This promotes subsequent osseous strength with the aid of the patient's own bone material, which is deposited during the operation. Patients who have an operation via posterior access can generally leave the clinic once the stitches have been taken out, no later than on the 14th day after the operation. What may be seen as a drawback to this procedure, however, is that the spine must be fused over a longer section than with anterior access.

The spine is thus more restricted in its overall mobility than when the anterior access method is used. There is usually freedom to choose between the two procedures with single-curve spinal curvature. In so-called "combined scoliosis" with very pronounced thoracic curvature and significant lumbar curvature, a posterior access operation or an operation from both the front and back promises greater success.

5.3.2 Anterior Access

Anterior access does not lie in the center of the trunk. As a rule, the incision is made along the ribs. One rib is removed, which, after being broken up into small pieces, is later inserted in the intervertebral spaces as the patient's own bone material for spanning purposes. Then, once the thoracic cavity and/or abdominal cavity is opened, the spine is exposed from the front (anterior). In this technique, the operating surgeon has free access to the vertebral bodies and intervertebral disks. For the corrective procedure, the intervertebral disks from the selected area are removed, and screws are inserted into the sides of the vertebral bodies being corrected. These screws are connected to a rod and, once correction is done, affixed to it. Taking the place of the removed intervertebral disks is the prepared bone material taken from the patient; in the lumbar region, this is sometimes additionally supported by small metal cages that are better able to maintain the space of the disk. This can prevent development of kyphosis (humpback) in the lumbar region. If the size of the vertebral body allows, modern surgical procedures implement two rods for better initial stability at the anterior access.

The anterior access operation has the disadvantage in that the abdominal and/or thoracic cavities have to be opened up. Even today, these operations sometimes require several months of post-operative brace treatment as well to secure the results. The indisputable benefit of the anterior procedure is that a smaller number of vertebral bodies are involved in the area being fused, meaning that better residual mobility and trunk function still remain after the operation.

Furthermore, a rib hump and lumbar protuberance can be almost completely eliminated with an anterior access operation directly after operation. A posterior access operation usually requires additional cosmetic surgery on the ribs to reduce the size of the rib hump.

The fact that the scar is concealed may well be regarded as yet another advantage of having an anterior access operation. It lies largely underneath the arm in the resting position and is not even visible when girls and women thus afflicted are seen from behind in bathing suits.

The operation according to Harrington was the first procedure with a rod using the posterior access method and was being applied worldwide by the end of the 1960s. The next innovative step came when Dwyer, an Australian, developed the anterior access operation, which Zielke then further developed as VDS, or "Ventral Derotation Spondylodesis." VDS has likewise been disseminated around the world.

The double rod systems that are now in use for posterior access were first introduced by Cotrel and Dubousset in 1984. This procedure has been globally applied since the end of the 1980s.

5.3.3 Current State of Development of Instruments Used for Scoliosis Correction

There are now more than 300 different implants available for spine-fusing operations. Today's wide array of implants makes it all but impossible to do justice to individual treatment principles theoretically or even practically, as is noted by Professor Heine in the foreword to the book "Die ventrale Instrumentation der Rumpfwirbelsäule" ("Ventral Instrumentation of the Trunk Spine") by P. Eysel (Enke-Verlag 1989).

The new developments do, however, have some advantages. Thanks to the new ventral double-rod systems, anterior access operations can now be performed without post-operative brace treatments. Furthermore, the fractures that occurred over time in the threaded rod of the original VDS are a thing of the past due to the durable rods currently being used. An example of the ventral (anterior) double-rod system is the Halm-Zielke instrument system, which allows the threaded rod to be reliably guided via a solid frame-plate that is fastened by two screws *(Fig. 5.33)*.

Figure 5.34 shows the radiological result of a 16-year-old girl with curvature straightening from 68° to 14° according to Cobb. The side profile was stretched as well, with the kyphosis that was more pronounced than normal in the

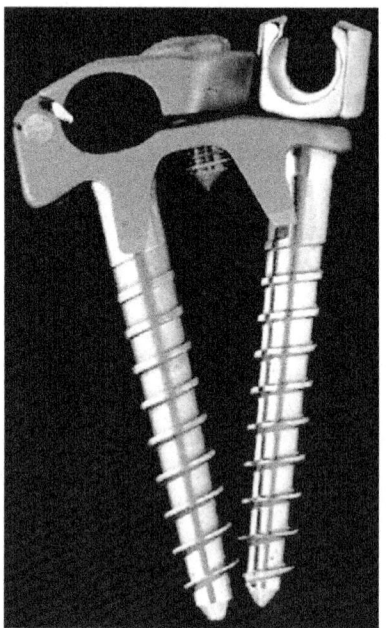

Fig. 5.33 The bracket of the Halm-Zielke instrumentation, which is fastened to the sides of the vertebrae with two screws (anterior access). A threaded rod and a solid profile rod are inserted through the holes in the screw head or the bracket, giving the instrumentation the necessary stability.

transitional area between the thoracic and lumbar spines being likewise straightened, as can be seen on the lateral images. Excellent treatment results without rib hump resection are clinically possible through three-dimensional form correction alone as well *(Fig. 5.35)*. It has even been possible to improve the correction options for posterior access surgical procedures by increasing the use of so-called pedicle screws. In *Figure 5.36*, you can see on the left the scoliosis of a 14-year-old girl with idiopathic combined scoliosis, which was able to be corrected almost completely through a posterior access operation.

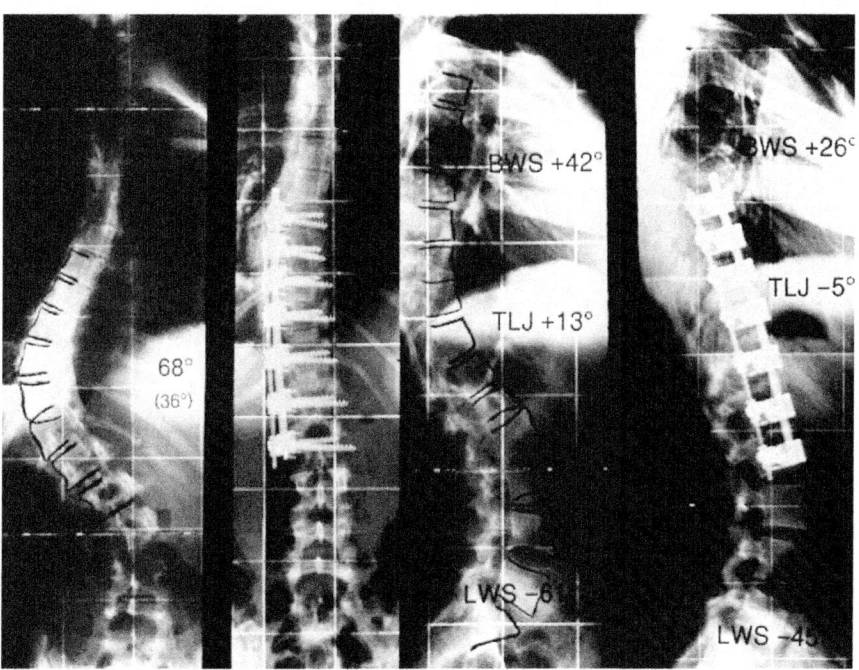

Fig. 5.34: A 16-year-old girl with idiopathic thoracolumbar scoliosis. Curvature straightening of 68° to 14° was achieved with the aid of the Halm-Zielke instrumentation, which also enabled the kyphosis clearly visible from the side to be partially straightened.

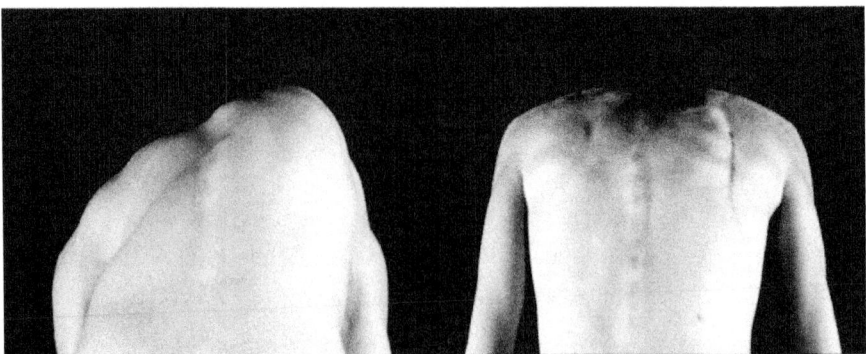

Fig. 5.35: Clinical picture of a 17-year-old boy before his operation (left) and afterwards (right). The rib hump has been completely rectified due to three-dimensional form correction, without further plastic surgery on the rib hump being necessary.

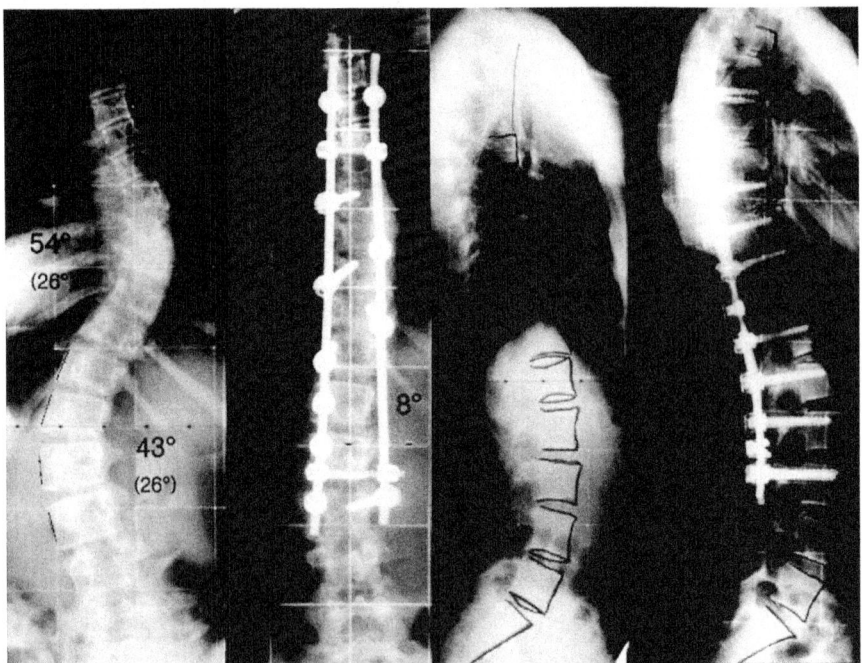

Fig. 5.36: A 14-year-old girl with idiopathic double-curve scoliosis. There was 54° in the thoracic area before the operation that was almost completely straightened afterwards with the use of so-called MPDS instrumentation via posterior spinal column access. The lateral profile of the spinal column was also positively affected by this operation.

Both anterior as well as posterior versions of this operation are standard procedure in the specialized spinal surgical centers of today. The choice of which operation is performed is solely determined by the extent of curvature, the curvature pattern, and the stiffness of the curvature, not by any limitation on the part of the surgeon.

These two surgical options are frequently used in combination for particularly stiff and severe curvatures. This means that it is possible to carry out ventral (anterior) straightening and additional dorsal (posterior) spondylodesis on the same day in a single operation, with the patients having to be turned during the procedure. *Figure 5.37* shows the X-ray with a curvature angle of 112° according to Cobb, which was able to be corrected to 28°. In this case, not only was the curvature straightened, but the result attained in the end was also very appealing from a cosmetic perspective.

More recent surgical procedures such as stapling described by *Betz* have not yet had any genuine indication. On the one hand, there are no long-term results available, and, on the other, the short to medium-term follow-ups show that this treatment procedure is not at all effective in curvatures beyond the 40° limit. Due to the fact that curvatures up to 40° and sometimes even greater, as shown above, can be excellently improved with currently standard braces and that this kind of treatment has been increasingly less likely to involve significant impairment, this form of operation needs to be viewed with suspicion[28] and cannot be recommended. Nevertheless, an ambitious marketing campaign was launched not long ago even in this part of the world.[29] In a more recent study concerning stapling, it was demonstrated that, within 2 years after an initial operation, about half of the patients had to be re-operated on.[30] It is thus clear that this procedure has not yet been perfected.

---

[28] Hans-Rudolf Weiss (2011) Treatment was uncritically reported. Dtsch Arztebl Int 108: 11. 189; author reply 189–189; author reply 190 Mar
http://www.aerzteblatt.de/v4/archiv/artikel.asp?id =81308

[29] Trobisch P, Suess O, Schwab F: Idiopathic Scoliosis. Dtsch Arztebl Int 2010; 107(49): 875–84. DOI: 10.3238/arztebl.2010.0875

[30] O'leary PT, Sturm PF, Hammerberg KW, Lubicky JP, Mardjetko SM. Convex hemiepiphysiodesis: the limits of vertebral stapling. Spine (Phila Pa 1976). 2011 Sep 1;36(19):1579-83.

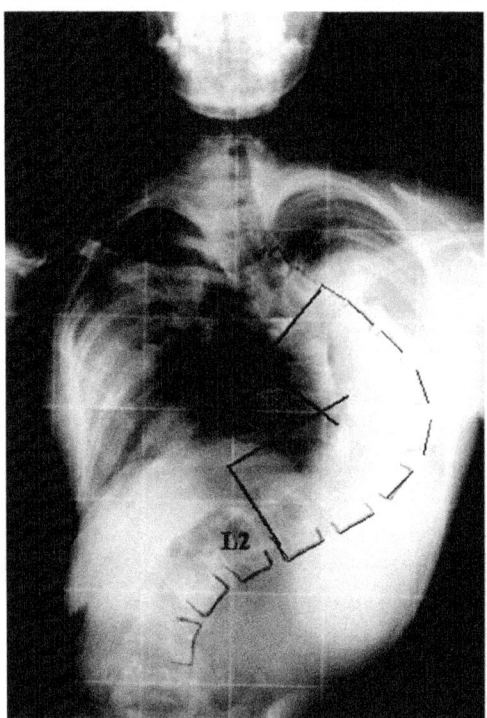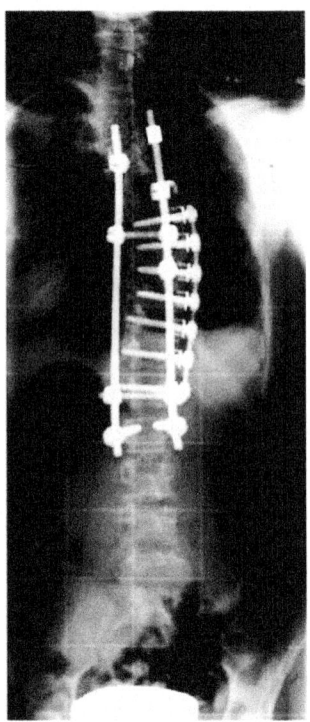

Fig. 5.37: Severe spinal curvature of 112° before the operation, performed combining both the anterior and posterior access methods on the same day. Straightening to 28° is considerable and out of the question if only one of the two forms of instrumentation is used.

In summary, we can state that the anterior access operation is more cosmetically pleasing and less functionally inhibiting option. Today it can be guaranteed that a posterior access operation can be performed without the need for a brace. Admittedly, it does not offer such favorable cosmetic results without additional rib-hump correction.

The overall short-term risk quoted for an operation to treat idiopathic scoliosis is about 5%. That means that 95% of the patients operated on can leave the hospital without any complications whatsoever, usually after no more than 14 days. The complications – in about 5% of the operations – can be broken down into:

- inflammations, which can generally be controlled by antibiotics,
- adverse respiratory effects due to postoperative bleeding, which can generally be alleviated with suitable suction drainage,
- rod or hook tear or rod fracture, necessitating follow-up surgery,
- or nervous disorders (less than 1%). In most cases, post-operative paralysis goes away again, and only a handful of patients can expect to have lasting nerve damage.

In major surgical centers, the operation risks appear to be low. They usually state that no cases of nerve damage from scoliosis operations have been determined in the last five to seven years.

This means that operations to treat idiopathic scoliosis can be regraded as having relatively few complications in the short term. However, the international literature has reported on the possibility of post-surgery pain occurring several years or even decades later, as well as a not insignificant number of patients requiring repeated follow-up surgery due to late complications. A fairly recent publication containing the long-term results of the Cotrel-Dubousset procedure reported that practically 50% of the patients had to undergo another operation within 20 years.[31] From the latest overview studies, it is slowly becoming clear that afflicted persons tend to suffer far more problems down the road after an operation than by going untreated.[32,33]

A medical indication for spinal fusion surgery in patients with scoliosis does not exist. This has been found in two Cochrane reviews (unbiased reviews

---

[31] Mueller FJ, Gluch H. Cotrel-dubousset instrumentation for the correction of adolescent idiopathic scoliosis. Long-term results with an unexpected high revision rate. Scoliosis. 2012;7(1):13. doi: 10.1186/1748-7161-7-13.

[32] Weiss HR, Moramarco M. Scoliosis – treatment indications according to current evidence. OA Musculoskeletal Medicine 2013 Mar 01;1(1):1.

[33] Weiss HR, Moramarco M, Moramarco K. Risks and long-term complications of adolescent idiopathic scoliosis surgery vs. non-surgical and natural history outcomes. Hard Tissue 2013 Apr 30;2(3):27.

guided by the Cochrane collaboration)[34,35] and in other systematic reviews as well.[36,37]

Additionally patients should be aware of the fact that the corrections as achieved by spinal fusion surgery are not necessarily stable *(Fig. 5.38)*.

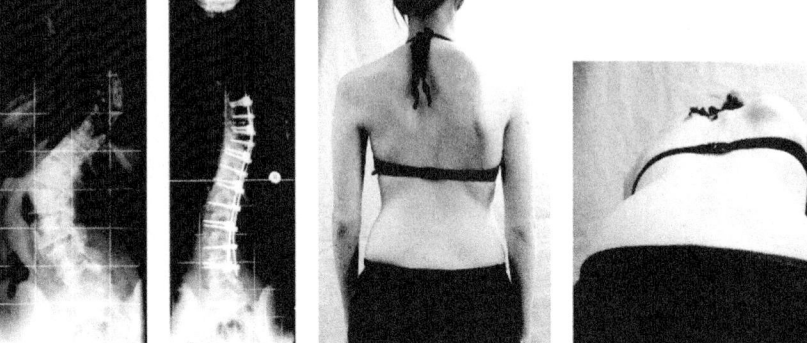

Fig. 5.38: Late result after spinal fusion surgery. The correction as achieved in the x-ray *(left)* can be regarde as being good, however, the ribhump 5 years after surgery has reappeared *(right)*.

---

[34] Bettany-Saltikov J, Weiss HR, Chockalingam N, Taranu R, Srinivas S, Hogg J, et al. Surgical versus non-surgical interventions in people with adolescent idiopathic scoliosis. Cochrane Database Syst Rev. 2015;4:CD010663.
[35] Cheuk DK, Wong V, Wraige E, Baxter P, Cole A. Surgery for scoliosis in Duchenne muscular dystrophy. Cochrane Database Syst Rev. 2015;10:CD005375.
[36] Weiss HR, Turnbull D, Tournavitis N, Borysov M (2016) Treatment of Scoliosis- Evidence and Management (Review of the Literature). Middle East J Rehabil Health.2016;3: epub ahead of print 2. April.
[37] Weiss HR, Goodall D. The treatment of adolescent idiopathic scoliosis (AIS) according to present evidence. A systematic review. Eur J Phys Rehabil Med. 2008;44(2):177-93.

6 What Restrictions Do I Have to Expect?

6.1 Scoliosis and Sports

General exemption from school sports for children and adolescents with scoliosis is not based on science. Sporting activities can also improve the performance of school-aged children and adolescents with scoliosis.

In a study by the Münster University Clinic, 150 patients with idiopathic scoliosis were examined. 100 of these patients, who had scoliosis from 10 to 50 degrees according to Cobb, participated in all sports activities offered by school and recreational athletics programs. 50 patients were generally exempted from sports. In 70-75% of the cases, there was no further increase in curvature – both in the group participating in school sports as well as in the control group – even though sports involving jolts to the spine were not excluded. For this reason, the authors spoke against general sports exemption. Their argument that exempting those affected by scoliosis from school sports shunts them into a psychologically disadvantaged outsider role merits consideration.

Although it is generally advised to take off braces during school sports, many leisure activities can also be enjoyed while wearing the brace without any substantial interference. In particular, the more recent brace varieties made with less material often permit a greater range of motion that only minimally gets in the way of the leisure activities of young people *(Figs. 6.1 a–b)*.

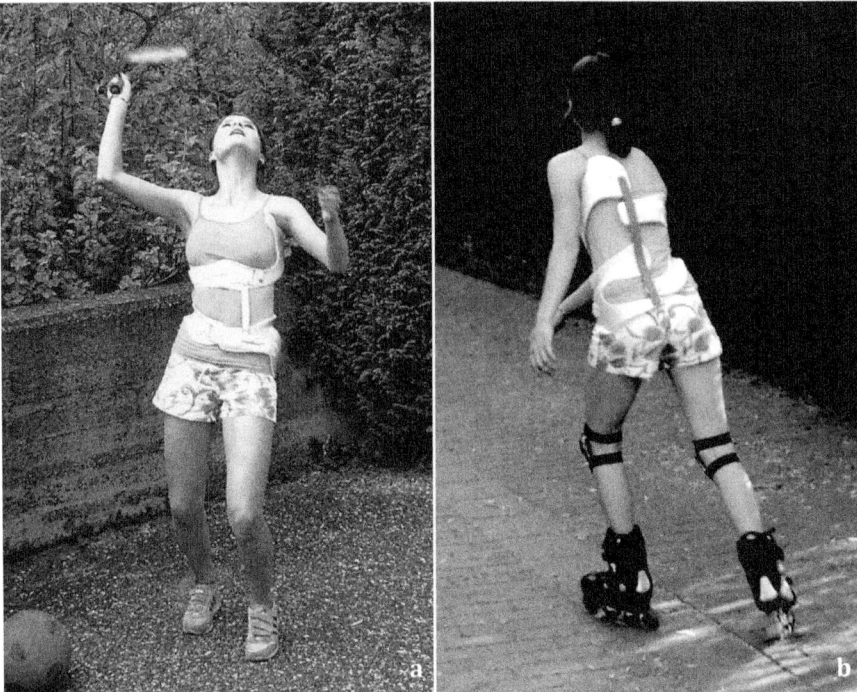

Figs. 6.1 a–b: A female patient with idiopathic scoliosis in a Chêneau light brace. She does not feel significantly restricted by the brace in her leisure time activities (© T. F. Müller).

6.2 Scoliosis and Pregnancy

As a rule, scoliosis is not negatively affected by pregnancy. A Swedish study attests that female patients with several pregnancies prior to their 23rd year can expect a greater chance of curvature increase. This is why it is recommended to avoid pregnancy before the end of the third decade of life. This is especially true for women who have been treated with a brace.

An Italian study also shows no systematic curvature increase during pregnancy. However, this study revealed that regular physical therapy during pregnancy arrests progredient scoliosis. In the study, of the women who had an initial angle of scoliosis exceeding 50 degrees, those who did not participate in regular physical therapy were most likely affected by a curvature increase after their third pregnancy.

From an obstetric point of view, there are no known long-term repercussions of scoliosis on pregnancy or the birth process. However, this is not always the case for women who have undergone a scoliosis operation. When there is a long fused section extending to the sacrum, the flexibility of the pelvic ring may well be reduced. Before planning a pregnancy, this topic should be discussed as a precaution with the surgeon performing the scoliosis operation as well as with a gynecologist, even though we are not aware of there ever having been any postoperative impediments to birth.

6.3 Scoliosis and Osteoporosis

In principle, bone density decreases in all people as they become older. This normal bone depletion process affects everyone at a certain age. Women in particular are affected by reduced calcium salt content early on after menopause. Then there is osteoporosis, which involves a greater than normal reduction in bone substance and thus requires treatment. Experience shows that scoliosis patients are very afraid of osteoporosis. It is common for the normal reduction in bone substance to be mistaken for pathological osteoporosis.

If humpback in a woman without scoliosis increases in the ten years after menopause, this should not be considered a pathological process. Progression of scoliosis at this age should not necessarily be regarded as pathological either.

It is a well-known phenomenon that slight curvatures that had previously stabilized on their own deteriorate at this age, which, however, does not mean that the affected person is more ill.

In treating "bone deficit," there is widespread agreement that using the axial organ, that is to say daily movement, significantly retards bone depletion. For this reason, movement in general, physical therapy, and inpatient rehabilitation are to be recommended at this age.

Dietary recommendations made for pathological osteopenia are, however, controversial. On the one hand, it is recommended that calcium intake be increased[38,39] and that more milk products be consumed to cover calcium requirements. On the other, it is known that too great an intake of protein will lead to increased calcium excretion. Thus the recommended foodstuffs, a large percentage of which are made up of protein, will probably lead to greater calcium excretion and might not help at all in the end.

A study from Boston,[40] according to which an increase in milk or cheese consumption in no way protects against the occurrence of dreaded bone fractures, is indicative of this problem. It goes so far as to state the opinion that osteoporosis may actually be triggered by milk products.[41] In any case, milk products must also be used with caution, because they may produce allergies in adults.[42] Furthermore, it has been proven that certain foodstuffs impair the intake of calcium from food, namely phosphatic sausage products, processed cheese and cola beverages, as well as vegetables containing oxalic acid. It has been discovered that the habitual consumption of cola drinks increases the bone fracture rate in school-age children.[43]

Traditional Chinese Medicine (TCM) disapproves of the beverages mentioned above and also of using milk products for treating osteoporosis. According to

---

[38] Ringe JD (Hrsg.) (1991) Osteoporose. Pathogenese, Diagnostik, Therapiemöglichkeiten. Walter de Gruyter, Berlin, New York

[39] Ziegler R (1990) Was ist gesichert in der Therapie der Osteoporose? Internist 31: 680–688

[40] Freskanich D, Willett WC, Stampfer MJ, Golditz GA (1977) Milk, dietary calcium and bone fractures in women: a 12-year prospective study. In: Am J Public Health 1997 Jun 87 (6): 992-997

[41] Runow KD (1997) Neue diagnostische Möglichkeiten bei multipler Chemikalien-Sensibilität (MCS) und chronischem Erschöpfungssyndrom (CFS): Umweltchemikalien, Zahnmetalle, Nahrungsallergene und Pilze. Vortrag auf dem XII. Internationalen Symposium für Umweltmedizin, Bad Ems, 5–7 September 1997

[42] Pollmer U (1997) Krank durch "gesunde Ernährung": Gesundheitsrisiken durch Getreide und Milch. Vortrag auf dem XII. Internationalen Symposium für Umweltmedizin. Bad Ems, 5–7 September 1997

[43] Petridou E, Karpathios T, Somou E, Trichopoulos D (1997) The role of dairy products and non-alcoholic beverages in bone fractures among schoolage children. In: Scand J Soc Med., Jun 25 (2): 119-125

the principles of Chinese medicine, these products cool down the spleen to such an extent that weariness, difficulty concentrating, and impaired digestion are the result.[44]

Now there is scientific evidence that adult scoliosis patients have below-average bone density. The extent to which these findings possess pathological significance, however, is not yet sufficiently clear.

6.4 What Do I Have to Expect in Old Age?

6.4.1 Pain

This is another question that concerns many patients with various curvature severity. For one thing, it is emphasized over and over again that the pain caused by scoliosis increases with age. This presumption is wrong. Pain and curvature angle are not dependent on each other. For another, there is a positive correlation between age and pain incidence, just as with non-scoliotic people. Therefore, there is no indication for patients without pain to be operated on in order to prevent future complaints of pain. I have encountered some patients with curvatures greater than 100 degrees who even beyond their 70th year never experienced pain as well as a few patients with rather low-degree curvatures suffering from pain that could hardly be ameliorated.

6.4.2 Cardiovascular Problems

Frequently, there are also fears with regard to possible restrictions in cardiovascular function. Such restrictions are possible. They usually occur only in curvatures beyond the 100 degree limit. For curvatures below 90 degrees, it is extremely likely that there will not be any serious performance restrictions. While it is true that curvatures below 90 degrees involve functional restrictions in the cardiovascular system that may be a burden at times, they can be treated successfully with a conservative approach. The prognosis concerning performance restrictions in adults and also in old age

---

[44] Flaws B, Wolfe HL (1995) Das Yin und das Yang der Ernährung. Das Handbuch der chinesischen Ernährungslehre. 3rd ed., Scherz Verlag Bern, München, Wien

depends on the location of the curvature, on the type and origin of the scoliosis, as well as on a few other factors. Accordingly, such a prognosis can only be assessed in an individual doctor-patient consultation.

The fear of a shortened lifespan needs to be dispelled in patients with curvatures in excess of 100 degrees as well. The statements included above are based on statistics from scientific investigations. However, they are not always pertinent in individual cases. Still, it can be concluded that, in light of the scientific findings described, existing or potential curvature angles greater than 90 degrees are an indication for an operation.

Finally, it must be emphasized that fears need to be vigorously dispelled in the course of talks with the attending doctors. Patients with moderate-degree curvature should not worry about being severely restricted in old age or bound to a wheelchair. This is not to be expected merely due to moderate scoliosis without severe accompanying illnesses.

6.5 Scoliosis and the Psyche

The psychological effects suffered by scoliosis patients are widely varied. Some are profoundly depressed by the diagnosis. Others are completely focused on finding a way of managing scoliosis on their own. In any event, the mental reactions are very distinct, as is evident from the patient reports.

Particularly during the developmental age, scoliosis may produce psychological problems due to the cosmetic changes. But even adults may be severely affected mentally, even if the complaints and curvatures are only moderate. From a statistical perspective, there is no correlation between the severity of scoliosis and psychosocial impairment. Many patients with minimal curvatures suffer from adverse mental effects, while others with very severe scoliosis appear only slightly affected. In one study on the topic of scoliosis and the psyche, we discovered that our adolescent and young-adult patients appeared more depressed compared to a control group. The study showed that their self-esteem and zest for life were reduced to a significant degree. What is more, contrary to expectations, the depression rate was higher for male participants in the study than for those that were female. Self-esteem and a positive attitude towards life had plummeted, with a clearly heightened tendency to focus on the problem. The question as to whether these changes are triggered by scoliosis or possibly even favor development of scoliosis has yet to be clarified.

7 Guidelines: Indication for Treating Cases of Scoliosis (status 6 / 2013)

The version of the guideline "Indication for the Conservative Treatment of Scoliosis" described below and adapted for Germany stems from in-depth consultations with international specialists in the field of conservative scoliosis treatment and from the basis for discussion presented during the SOSORT Conference in Milan and the original work published in 2006 (Hans-Rudolf Weiss, Stefano Negrini, Manuel Rigo, Tomasz Kotwicki, Martha C Hawes, Theodoros B Grivas, Toru Maruyama, Franz Landauer (2006) **Indications for Conservative Management of Scoliosis (guidelines).** *Scoliosis* 1: 05). The subsequent review in the 2011 SOSORT guidelines resulted in more complexity without significant changes to the content, however, the latter guidelines have the drawback that the treatment method being looked up is rather difficult to find.

Definition

Scoliosis is defined as a lateral curvature of the spine with torsion of the spine and chest, as well as a disturbance of the sagittal profile.

Etiology

Idiopathic scoliosis is the most common of all forms of lateral deviation of the spine. By definition, it is a lateral curvature of the spine in an otherwise healthy child for which a recognizable cause has not been found. Recent investigations have focussed on a functional tethering of the spinal cord or neuro-osseus disturbance, which may result in a ventral overgrowth; however, loss of lumbar lordosis has not yet been clearly explained. Less common but better defined etiologies of the disorder include scoliosis of neuromuscular origin, congenital scoliosis, scoliosis in neurofibromatosis,

Prader Willi syndrome, and mesenchymal disorders such as Marfan's syndrome.

Epidemiology

The prevalence of adolescent idiopathic scoliosis (AIS), when defined as a curvature greater than 10° according to Cobb, is 2-3%. The prevalence of curvatures greater than 20° is between 0.3 and 0.5%, while curvatures greater than 40° according to Cobb are found in less than 0.1% of the population. All etiologies of scoliosis other than AIS are encountered more rarely.

Classifications

The anatomical level of the deformity has received attention from clinicians as a basis for scoliosis classification. The level of the apex vertebra (i.e. thoracic, thoracolumbar, lumbar, or double major) forms a simple basis for description. In 1983 King and colleagues classified different curvature patterns by the extent of spinal fusion required; however, recent reports have suggested that these classifications lack reliability. Another description has been developed by Lenke and colleagues. This approach calls for clinical assessment of scoliosis and kyphosis with respect to sagittal profile and curvature components. Systems designed for conservative management include the classifications by Lehnert-Schroth (functional three-curve and functional four-curve scoliosis) and recently by Weiss (used for brace construction and application).

Objectives of Conservative Management

The primary goal of scoliosis management is to stop curvature progression. Improving pulmonary function (vital capacity) and treating pain are also of major importance. The first of two methods of conservative scoliosis management is based on physical therapy, including Méthode Lyonaise, Side Shift, Schroth, "Best Practice," and others. Although discussed from contrasting viewpoints in the international literature, today there is evidence for the effectiveness of scoliosis treatment using physical therapy alone.

It has to be emphasised that (1) physical therapy for scoliosis does not just consist of general exercises, but rather one of the cited methods designed to address the particular nuances of spinal deformity, and (2) the application of such methods requires that therapists and clinicians be specifically trained and certified in these scoliosis-specific conservative intervention methods.

Scoliosis intensive rehabilitation (SIR), which once appeared at least in short-term to be effective in regard to many signs and symptoms of scoliosis and with respect to impeding curvature progression, seems outdated today in view of the fact that outpatient therapies can produce the same results. Initially a 6-week intensive inpatient program was investigated; however, the results achieved in this outdated setting cannot effectively be compared to the results of today's programs with reduced rehabilitation times and modified programs. More intensive outpatient programs are provided that does not seem less effective than the current inpatient program.[45,46,47]

The second mode of conservative management is brace treatment, which has been found to be effective in preventing curvature progression and thus in altering the natural history of IS. It appears that brace treatment may reduce the prevalence of surgery, restore the sagittal profile and influence vertebral rotation. There are also indications that the end result of brace treatment can be predicted. Currently this applies to hard bracing only. Independent studies on soft braces have shown that there is no indication for the use of such devices.

---

[45] HR Weiss, S Seibel (2010) Scoliosis Short-Term Rehabilitation (SSTR) – A Pilot Investigation, The Internet Journal of Rehabilitation. 1: 1. 11

[46] Borysov M, Borysov A. Scoliosis short-term rehabilitation (SSTR) according to 'Best Practice' standards-are the results repeatable? Scoliosis. 2012 Jan 17;7(1):1. doi: 10.1186/1748-7161-7-1.

[47] Pugacheva N. Corrective exercises in multimodality therapy of idiopathic scoliosis in children - analysis of six weeks efficiency - pilot study. Stud Health Technol Inform. 2012;176:365-71.

Systematic Application of the Two Methods of Conservative Treatment with Respect to Cobb Angle and Maturity

Guidelines for conservative intervention are based on current information regarding the risk for significant curvature progression in a given period of time. Each case has its own natural history and must be considered on an individual basis in the context of a thorough clinical evaluation and patient history. Estimation of risk for progression is based on epidemiological surveys in which children diagnosed with scoliosis were radiographed periodically to quantify changes in curvature magnitude over time. Such surveys support the premise that, among populations of children with a diagnosis of idiopathic scoliosis, the risk of progression is highly correlated with potential for growth over the period of observation. In boys the prognosis for progression is more favourable, with relatively fewer individuals having curves that progress to >40 degrees. For the German guidelines, prognostic risk estimation is based on the calculation of Lonstein and Carlson. This calculation is based on curvature progression observed among 727 patients (575 female, 152 male) diagnosed between 1974 and 1979 in school screening programs in the State of Minnesota (United States) and followed until they reached skeletal maturity.

I. Children (no signs of maturity)

a. Cobb angle <15°: Observation (6-12 month intervals).

b. Cobb angle 15–20°: Physical therapy with treatment-free intervals (6-12 weeks without physical therapy for those patients having low risk for curve progression at the time).

c. Cobb angle 20–25°: Physical therapy.

d. Cobb angle >25°: Physical therapy and brace wearing (part-time, 12-16 hours).

II. Children and adolescents, Risser 0–3, first signs of maturation, less than 98% of mature height

The following section is based on progression risk rather than on Cobb angle measurement because of the changing risk profiles for deformity as the skeleton matures. For our purposes, progression risk is calculated by the formula shown in *Fig. 7.1*.

a. *Progression risk <40%: Observation (3-month intervals).*

b. *Progression risk 40%: Physical therapy.*

c. *Progression risk 60%: Physical therapy + part-time brace indication (16-23 hours [low risk]).*

d. *Progression risk 80%: Physical therapy + full-time brace indication (23 hours [high risk]).*

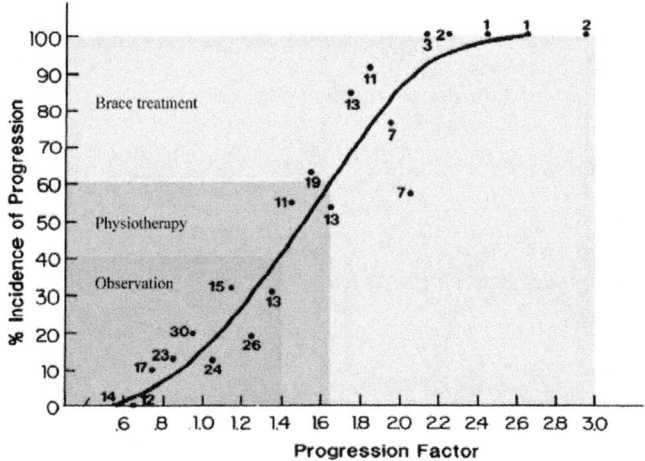

Graph showing the incidence of progression according to the progression factor, which is calculated by the formula:

$$\frac{\text{Cobb angle} - (3 \times \text{Risser stage})}{\text{Chronological age}} = \text{Progression factor}$$

Fig. 7.1: The illustration shows the incidence of the progression according to the progression factor, calculated using the formula: Cobb angle − (3 x Risser sign) / chronological age. (modified from Lonstein and Carlson)

III. Children and adolescents presenting with Risser 4 (more than 98% of mature height)

a. Cobb angle <20°: Observation (6-12 month intervals).

b. Cobb angle 20-35°: Physical therapy.

c. Cobb angle >35°C: Physical therapy + brace (part-time, about 16 hours are sufficient).

d. For brace weaning: Physical therapy + brace with reduced wearing time.

IV. First presentation with Risser 4–5 (more than 99.5% of mature height before growth is completed)

a. Cobb angle >25°: Physical therapy.

b. Cobb angle >35°: Physical therapy + brace (part-time, about 16 hours are sufficient in cosmetic indication only, when surgery can be avoided).

V. Adults with Cobb angles >30°

Physical therapy, inpatient rehabilitation.

VI. Adolescents and adults with scoliosis (of any degree) and chronic pain

Physical therapy, scoliosis rehabilitation program

(multimodal pain concept/behavioral + physical concept),

brace treatment when a positive effect has been proven during specific testing.

The prognostic estimation and corresponding indications for treatment apply to the most prevalent condition: idiopathic scoliosis. In other types of scoliosis a similar procedure can be applied. Exceptions include cases where the prognosis is clearly worse, for example in neuromuscular scoliosis where a wheelchair is necessary (surgery for maintaining sitting capability may be required). Other reasons for considering alternative treatments include:

- *Severe decompensation*
- *Severe sagittal deviations with structural lumbar kyphosis ("flatback")*
- *Lumbar, thoracolumbar, and caudal component of double curvatures with a disproportionate rotation compared to the Cobb angle and with a high risk of future instability at the caudal junctional zone*
- *Severe contractures and muscle shortening*
- *Reduced mobility of the spine, especially in the sagittal plane*
- *Others to be individually considered.*

Definition of Terms:

Physiotherapy: The indication of physiotherapy during the main growth spurt is only relative. Since in the case of patients who do not receive treatment during the main growth spurt, some 30% remain without a change for the worse, 50% after several inpatient treatments (according to results from the end of the 1980s), 70% with treatment using the Boston brace without physiotherapy, and 80% with the old Chêneau brace, brace treatment is indicated absolutely and paramountly *(Fig. 7.2)*. Outside of the main growth spurt, physiotherapy can, however, be effective by itself.

The one and only reason for implementing today's inpatient measures or more intensive physiotherapy during the main growth spurt is the psychological effect, although inpatient rehabilitation measures are the preferred method for scoliosis patients with pain or lung function impairment. With a favorable prognosis or with brace treatment, two to five 90-minute sessions or one short outpatient rehabilitation of several days are often all that is necessary for acquiring the skills needed for the home exercise program. This does, however, presuppose that the therapy measures are of good quality and that the latest methods are being used.

Inpatient rehabilitation is prescribed for patients with chronic complaints.

Brace: In contrast to moderate braces (Boston brace, 70% not progressive), the old Chêneau brace (status 1999) had a proven success quota of 80% *(see Fig. 7.2)*. According to the latest scientific findings, the success quota of the most recent brace design (Chêneau-Gensingen®) lies at over 95%, with the curvature angle generally improving when there is a full-time wearing period and clear residual growth.

Short-term scoliosis rehabilitation programs are now being tested for both outpatient as well as inpatient treatment. Initial positive results are already available. For the very latest concepts that take the daily routine (Activities of daily living) into account (Scoliologic® Best Practice Program), it is more a question of changing the postural habits in everyday life. If this is successful after a short rehabilitation period and if the newly corrected postural patterns can successfully become automatic, further physiotherapy can be done without. This program would interfere with patients the least.

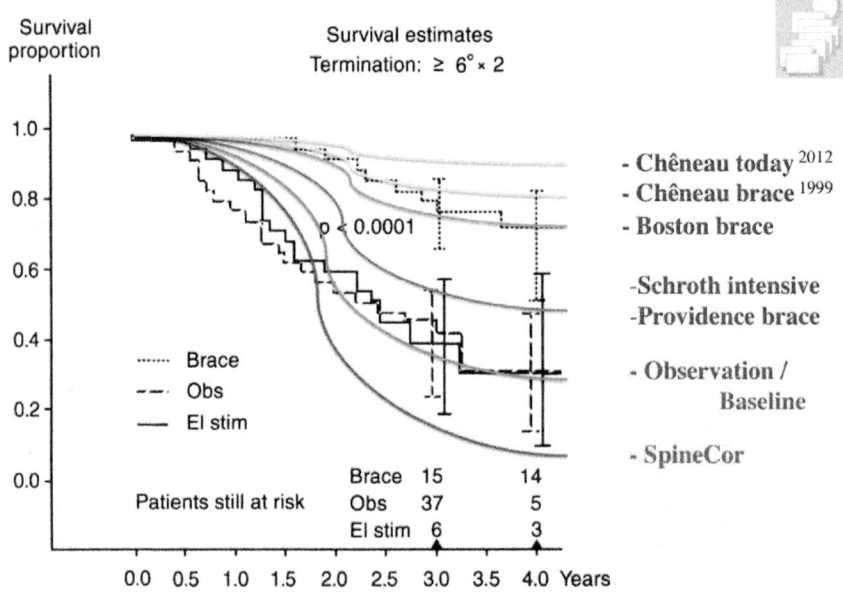

Fig. 7.2 Survival analysis (survival rate = statistical description for the number of non-progredient cases) of different treatment procedures during the main growth spurt. The "survival proportion" describes the proportion of non-progredient cases, in other words the cases where curvature has not increased. Without treatment 0.3 (30% without curvature increase), intensive inpatient Schroth therapy 0.5 (50% without curvature increase), Boston brace without physiotherapy in the USA 0.7 (70% without curvature increase), standard Chêneau brace after a plaster cast in 1999, sometimes with physiotherapy (80% without curvature increase), Chêneau-Gensingen brace CAD / CAM (>95% without curvature increase).

8 Summary

Central to the observations made in this guidebook is scoliosis of unknown origin, which we call idiopathic. Many matters described here can also be used for scoliosis of known cause. The forms of scoliosis of known cause are, however, so rare and the causes so diverse that they could not be described systematically in a guidebook such as this. Accordingly, consultation in these cases can only take the individual conditions into consideration. For this reason, general statements are not able to be made on this topic. And yet, what also applies to non-idiopathic scoliosis is that it may deteriorate in periods of bone growth, and cardiovascular problems may crop up in scoliosis cases in excess of 90 degrees in the thoracic region.

Idiopathic scoliosis (70-90% of all forms of scoliosis are idiopathic) only harbors major health risks in a few cases.

While it is true that during adulthood performance may be reduced with major curvatures, it can, however, be improved once again by rehabilitation measures at a suitable center or even by intensifying physical activities. Curvature deterioration can be usually be halted by selective procedures up until menopause, even for major curvatures.

It is my hope that this book achieves my objective: for one thing, disclosing treatment requirements to my readers, and for another, portraying the situation in such a defused manner that the understandable fears can subside. Overall, this guidebook is also meant to provide support for physicians, chiropractors, physical therapists and orthopedic technicians to enable them to calm their patients' fears during treatment and confidently present the merits of their effective treatment measures.

Extensive literature references are generally not the norm in a guidebook. It is certainly not necessary for lay people to read the specialist literature. It can, however, be helpful for those afflicted to know that certain claims are supported by a host of scientific studies. For this reason, I have made a list in the annex of the literature this book is based on, adding particularly important literature as footnotes, in the hopes that these extensive references will prove helpful for alleviating any uncertainty.

I would like to express my gratitude to the many patients whose questions motivated me to prepare this guidebook and, above all, to those who have enriched this little book with their personal reports. Many thanks indeed to all those patients who worked through this guidebook critically beforehand, thereby providing valuable assistance. I would also like to thank Prof. Dr. Halm for his critical tips, as well as for providing me with the photographs of surgically treated scoliosis patients.

The author wishes to acknowledge that this book is <u>not</u> meant to replace a presentation in the office of a physician specialized in spinal deformity treatment!

Conservative specialists

Below are addresses of conservative specialists where patients may receive advice according to the current protocols with respect to the conservative management of scoliosis. It is advisable to schedule a consultation in order to allow clinical / radiological investigation and initiate conservative treatment according to the most up-to-date standards.

Germany:

Hans-Rudolf Weiss, MD
Orthopedic Surgeon, Physical Medicine and Rehabilitation, Chiropractor (German school)
Alzeyer Str. 23
D-55457 Gensingen, Germany
Tel.: ++49 (0)6727 894040
Email: info@skoliose-dr-weiss.com
www.scoliosis-dr-weiss.com

USA:

Marc Moramarco, DC
Scoliosis 3DC
3 Baldwin Green Common
Suite 204
Woburn, MA 01801
781-938-8558
Email: info@scoliosis3dc.com
www.scoliosis3dc.com

Canada:

Fariba Taheri, PT
Best Practice Instructor
North York Total Rehabilitation
5292, Yonge Street, North York
Cell: 416 953 10 61
Email: faribataheri62@gmail.com

China:

Xiaofeng Nan, CPO
Official distributor Mainland China
(Physical Rehabilitation & Bracing) Orthotist,
Registered Schroth Best Practice Therapist
Nan Xiaofeng's Spinal Orthopedic Workshop
Beilin district of Xi 'an Shaanxi, China
http://www.haozhiju.com.
Email: nanxiaofeng19@gmail.com

Xiaofeng Nan, CPO
Official distributor Mainland China
(Physical Rehabilitation & Bracing) Orthotist,
Registered Schroth Best Practice Therapist
Room 1916 Park Cheer Residences, Bin Sheng Road No. 1870,
Binjiang District of Hangzhou, Zhejiang Province, Hangzhou
Email: nanxiaofeng19@gmail.com

Xie Hua, CPO
(Physical Rehabilitation & Bracing) Orthotist,
Registered Schroth Best Practice Therapist
in cooperation with *Nan Xiaofeng, CPO* (Official distributor Mainland China)
Luo Liping, PT (+86-13983885579; physical rehabilitation service)
Registered Schroth Best Practice Therapist
Room 2801, Building 4, Daping Vanke Center, No.160 Daping Street,
Yuzhong District, Chongqing city, China
Email:Xiehua:xiehuamail@163.com

Xie Hua, CPO
(Physical Rehabilitation & Bracing) Orthotist,
Registered Schroth Best Practice Therapist
in cooperation with *Nan Xiaofeng, CPO* (Official distributor Mainland China)
Room 1409, National Research Center for Rehabilitation Technical Aids,
Ronghua zhong Road No.1, Daxing District of Beijing

Prof. Dr. Tong Shen
(Physical Rehabilitation & Bracing),
Director of the Department of Rehabilitation, Distinguished chief expert,
Longjikang Spine Clinic (Guangzhou, China)
Dr. Huiling Du
(Physical Rehabilitation & Bracing),
Email: 228605437@qq.com
Tianming Xu, CPO
(Physical Rehabilitation & Bracing),
Email: 791341140@qq.com
The First Affiliated Hospital of Guangzhou Medical University,
Rehabilitation Specialist, Orthotist, Clinician,
Physiotherapist Orthopedic Rehabilitation Services.
Clinic Address: No.151, Yangtze River West Road,
Yuexiu District Province,Guangzhou, China
Or: Jinsui Road No.42,Zhujiang new town,
Tianhe district, Guangzhou, China
http://www.longjikang.com
Email: spine.cn@163.com

Cyprus:

Scoliosis Best Practice Rehab Services, Cyprus
(CEO: Nico Tournavitis)
Official distributor Greece & Cyprus
(Physical Rehabilitation & Bracing in cooperation with
Eleni Dracopoulou, PT, Schroth Therapist)
Conservative Treatment Center For Spinal Deformities
Michalakopoulou 14, 1075 Nicosia, Cyprus
Email : info@scoliosis-sbprs.com

Greece:

Scoliosis Best Practice Rehab Services, Thessaloniki
(CEO: Nico Tournavitis)
Official distributor Greece
(Physical Rehabilitation & Bracing
in cooperation with *Nikos Karavidas, PT*)
Conservative Treatment Center For Spinal Deformities
Aristotelous 5, GR 54624, Thessaloniki, Greece
Email: info@scoliosis-sbprs.com

Scoliosis Best Practice Rehab Services, Athens
(CEO: Nico Tournavitis)
Official distributor Greece
(Physical Rehabilitation & Bracing
in cooperation with *Nikos Karavidas, PT*)
Conservative Treatment Center For Spinal Deformities
10 Kifisias Ave. 11524 Athens, Greece
Email: info@scoliosis-sbprs.com

Hong Kong:

Dr. Shu Yan Ng, DC
Official distributor Hong Kong
(Physical Rehabilitation & Bracing) Chiropractor,
Registered Schroth Best Practice Therapist
1/fl China Hong Kong Tower, 8 Hennessy Road, Wanchai, Hong Kong
Email: ngshuyanhcc@gmail.com

Indonesia:

Dr. Budi S Widjaja, MD, QN
Official distributor Indonesia
Spine Clinic Family Holistic (Jakarta, Indonesia)
Scolisosis Rehabilitation Specialist, Acupuncture Specialist,
Cranial Functional Therapist, Registered Schroth Best Practice Therapist,
Orthopedic Rehabilitation Services,
Best Practice Bracing Center
http://www.bracetulangbelakang.com
Clinic Address: Jl. Daan Mogot 176A, Jakarta Barat, Indonesia 11520
Email: info@kliniktulangbelakang.com

Japan:

Yosuke Shiraishi, PhD
Chiiko Ishihara, JT
Schroth Best Practice Japan Inc.
Official distributor Japan
4-8-29 Kojimachi JP 0083, Tokyo, Japan
Email: yo.shirajp@gmail.com

Russia:

Mogiliantseva, Tatiana
City hospital №40
Borysova str. 9
Saint-Petersburg, Russia
Email: Tatiana_mog@mail.ru

South Korea:

Sang Gil (Daniel) Lee 이상길
Best Practice Instructor
Seoul
Email: whitesk79@nate.com

Ukraine:

Maksym Borysov
Best Practice Instructor
"Orttech-plus" Rehabilitation Services
Kharkiv (61037), Ukraine
www.schrothbestpractice.com.ua
Email: bma-ukrniip@mail.ru
          schroth-ukraine@ukr.net

Departments for physical rehabilitation worldwide apply the *Schroth Best Practice Program*:

https://schrothbestpractice.com/physical-rehabilitation-schroth-best-practice-standard/

Annex: Instructions for Use

Corrective Scoliosis Orthoses of the Chêneau Type for Scoliosis in Adolescence

Made to Specifications

You have received a corrective scoliosis orthosis that has been individually made for you by your specialist technical orthopedic service center. Please read through these instructions for use, which contain a great deal of important information and safety instructions.

Our team will be only too glad to answer any further questions you might have.

Important Information about Your Corrective Scoliosis Orthosis

Application and Restrictions for Use

Your scoliosis orthosis is designed to correct your scoliotically (three-dimensionally) changed spine. It uses truss pads to exercise pressure on certain parts of the body, pressure that has to spread to the clearance spaces on the opposite side to be relieved. Together with your exercises, your brace is meant to straighten the curvature of your spine and improve trunk statics. Wearing comfort and wearing duration of your scoliosis correction orthosis very largely depend on the severity, form, and location of your scoliosis, but also on your collaboration. What therapy result you will achieve with your scoliosis orthosis will depend on your individual clinical picture and overall constitution. As to whether accompanying therapeutic measures (e.g. physiotherapy) might help your performance, please discuss this with your attending doctor – likewise the daily wearing time.

Your corrective scoliosis orthosis should basically fit at all times without causing any complaints. Excessive pressure or chafe marks may lead to complications.

If you have any problems with your corrective scoliosis orthosis, please address them to your specialist technical orthopedic service center!

In order to maintain the function and reliability of your corrective scoliosis orthosis, it has to be treated with care. Any kind of excess strain or improper handling can lead to limited function or material failure: Your corrective orthosis is designed solely for the field of application determined with your doctor.

You are perfectly welcome to pursue sporting activities; however, choosing the kinds of sporting activities you engage in and how to go about this with your scoliosis orthosis should be discussed with your doctor, since your corrective scoliosis orthosis is not suitable for every sport. Using it in fresh and salt water and coming into contact with acids, lyes, and solvents should likewise be avoided. Exception: The orthosis is called "waterproof" and is expressly approved for cleaning with water, showering, and swimming.

You should not use your scoliosis orthosis at high temperatures, e.g. in the sauna, as the metal parts in contact with the skin may cause burns. High temperatures can lead to the plastic parts no longer fitting well.

Description of the Individual Components/Accessories

A scoliosis orthosis according to Chêneau is made of a rigid material that surrounds the trunk and fastens at the front. Furthermore, depending on the form of scoliosis, there are truss pads in different positions that exert a corrective force on the body. There should be clearance spaces opposite these truss pads where the pressure can escape to.

Medico-Therapeutic Aspects

Depending on your overall constitution and any existing accompanying illnesses, some complications may be incurred with your scoliosis brace on an individual basis. Address all problems involving your orthosis to your specialist technical orthopedic service center.

Your corrective scoliosis orthesis encircles the trunk and uses corrective truss pads to restraighten the deformed spine along different planes.

Each time you breathe in, your body has to move into these spaces in order to support passive correction.

Regular physical therapy is a good way to attain optimum corrective success. Your doctor can give you further tips concerning muscle training. Your corrective scoliosis orthosis is part of a therapy concept and can only have its ideal effect with your full cooperation. Keeping to the daily wearing time, the supervised physiotherapeutic exercises, and daily exercise at home are components of scientifically approved measures that contribute to success.

In addition to general personal hygiene, it is essential to observe the skin well, especially in the area of the truss pads. The permanent corrective pressure of the truss pads may cause changes to the skin color (redness). A dark-red, bluish discoloration or an open skin area is, however, not acceptable. In order to toughen up your skin, especially in these pressure zones, you can treat the areas by rubbing in skin-tanning agents such as PC 30 (which you can procure from your medical supply store). After showering or bathing, the skin must be completely dry again and not softened before you put your scoliosis orthosis back on.

Creams should generally be avoided, as they soften the skin, thereby making it less resistant to pressure.

Do not use any body powder, as this will chafe the skin under the truss pads and cause excessive dryness.

Direct contact of leather materials with injured skin must be avoided at all costs.

Handling / Functionality / Wearing-in of the Brace / Risks

Putting on and taking off the corrective scoliosis orthosis

You will have to learn how to handle your scoliosis orthosis, especially when you are receiving one for the first time. The act of putting it on and taking it off will take practice.

Your orthosis is not worn directly on the skin, but over a tight T-shirt or a brace shirt. This serves to more effectively bind or dissipate the moisture that forms under the brace. Take care to ensure that the shirt under the orthosis lies *wrinkle-free* on the skin to avoid unnecessary pressure marks. Even more suitable are special seamless brace shirts that are offered with sleeves. If needed, ask your orthopedic technician.

Since your scoliosis orthosis may well brings the lumbar spine and pelvis into a certain position, it is advisable to fasten it while lying on your back with legs slightly bent. It is easier in this position.

Please do not, however, pull the straps/closures *as tight as possible*, since the internal organs need more space when you are standing, and the brace will then be too tight. To sit up, roll on your side and push yourself up with your arms until you are sitting up.

Wearing Duration

The scoliosis orthosis made for you should be worn daily unless your doctor prescribes otherwise. The daily wearing time conforms to the degree value, the rigidity of your scoliosis, and with your current growth rate. Scoliosis orthoses generally should be worn for 23 hours (with one hour for personal hygiene) a day.

Getting Used to Wearing Your Brace

Once the trial fitting and initial changes for improving the wearing comfort of the brace have been carried out, it should be worn as long as possible. The wearing period of 23 hours a day should be attained as soon as possible.

Tip: After a meal, the brace can be opened a bit for about 20 to 30 minutes, but not taken off. Afterwards, the brace is properly re-closed.

Risks

The rigid brace construction will hamper you in certain movements. However, for the corrective forces to having an effect on your body, nothing can be done to avoid this.

Your corrective scoliosis brace is worn between your body and outerwear. This is why your clothing may show greater wear due to friction at the edges of the orthosis, while increased sweating may lead to skin irritations under the orthosis. If there are any changes to the skin, please consult your orthopedic technician or doctor.

Your scoliosis orthosis is a brace treatment prescribed during growth that provides a constant corrective effect. It is precisely because of this correction as well as normal physical growth in height and width that the brace may well become too small or the truss pads no longer be positioned properly. Keep tabs on the truss pad location and pressure as well as on your body size, and get in touch with your orthopedic technician as soon as you notice any change!

Special attention has been paid to the materials used for your scoliosis orthosis. As such, they have been tested for skin tolerance. Should changes to the skin nevertheless occur, consult your doctor promptly. Since your brace is made of plastic, possibly even metal and leather, it must not be subjected to direct flame or intense heat. It might catch fire or lose its shape.

Other medically significant risks are extremely rare. One case involving deep vein thrombosis of the leg is known that had to be treated with Marcumar. This was certainly not solely due to the front bottom edge of the brace pressing into the groin. There have to be other factors involved as well (basic illnesses, extreme dehydration after protracted sports activities, or the like) for leg vein thrombosis to occur during brace treatment. This kind of complication is not to be expected merely from wearing a brace.

Apart from growth-related changes to the curvature pattern, which need to be ruled out through the regular quarterly routine checkups, there are also occasional brace-induced cosmetic complications. In rare cases, chest development may be adversely affected if, with existing breast growth, the edge of the brace beneath the breast presses against the mammary gland for longer than 4 weeks.

In closing, however, it should be noted that such complications are extremely rare. After having approved or assessed more than 30,000 braces to date, the author has observed breast deformity complications a mere five times. These cases would have been avoidable if the patients concerned had paid attention and/or regularly gone to the routine checkups as prescribed.

Cleaning and Disinfecting the Brace

As with other clothing, your scoliosis orthosis also needs to be cleaned regularly to avoid unpleasant smells. The plastic or metal parts can washed off with water and soap. Leather parts should be wiped with a damp cloth from time to time. Washing would dry the leather and cause material failure.

As a rule, it is not necessary to disinfect the brace; however, it is advisable to do this from time to time if there are open or oozing wounds. To do so, it is sufficient to spray the contact surfaces with 70% isopropanol solution, 3% hydrogen peroxide solution, or other commercial disinfectants. It is possible that disinfection would cause colored braces, Velcro® fasteners, etc. to fade. If there is a leather truss pad, it could likewise be dried out by disinfectants.

Inspection and Maintenance

Your scoliosis orthosis must be checked regularly to ensure that proper fit and function is being maintained. Please be sure to observe the maintenance intervals in any event. Therefore, pay close attention to the maintenance intervals.
If you do not stick to the maintenance intervals, this will limit and possibly even nullify the liability of the specialist technical orthopedic service center should there be any damage.

Liability only covers the product if it retains the form it had when we delivered it. It extends only to services performed by the specialist technical orthopedic service center.

Disposal and Environmental Protection

In accordance with our activities for environmental protection, we would ask you to hand over your scoliosis orthosis to the specialist technical orthopedic service center for disposal.

Other remarks:

_____

_____

_____

Service life of the brace: It depends on your individual height and width growth.

Maintenance interval: After consultation with your doctor – generally three months.

(Based on the standards of the Federal Association of Orthopedic Technology)

Your specialist orthopedic service center:

Literature

Appelgren G, Willner S (1990). End Vertebra Angle – A Roentgenographic Method to Describe a Scoliosis. A Follow-up Study of Idiopathic Scoliosis Treated with the Boston Brace. *Spine* 15:71–74.

Berman AT, Cohen DL, Schwentker EP (1982). The effects of pregnancy on idiopathic scoliosis: A preliminary report on eight cases and review of literature. *Spine* 7:76.

Bettany-Saltikov J, Weiss HR, Chockalingam N, Taranu R, Srinivas S, Hogg J, et al. Surgical versus non-surgical interventions in people with adolescent idiopathic scoliosis. *Cochrane Database Syst Rev.* 2015;4:CD010663.

Blount WP, Mellencamp DD (1980). The effect of pregnancy on idiopathic scoliosis. *J Bone Joint Surg Am* 62:1083.

Borysov M, Borysov A. (2012). Scoliosis short-term rehabilitation (SSTR) according to 'Best Practice' standards-are the results repeatable? *Scoliosis* Jan 17;7(1):1. doi: 10.1186/1748-7161-7-1.

Bös K, Wydra G, Karisch G (1992). Gesundheitsförderung durch Bewegung, Spiel und Sport. Perimed-Fachbuch-Verlag.-Ges., Erlangen.

Brooks HL, Azen SP, Gerberg EI et al. (1975). Scoliosis: a prospective epidemiological study. *J Bone Joint Surg Am* 57:968.

Bundesverband der Ärzte für Orthopädie e.V. (BVO). Osteoporose – Ein Leitfaden für Patienten. Bezugsadresse: Am Lindenbaum 6–8, 60433 Frankfurt/M.

Bunnell WP (1986). A study of the natural history of idiopathic scoliosis before skeletal maturity. *Spine* 11:773.

Cheuk DK, Wong V, Wraige E, Baxter P, Cole A. Surgery for scoliosis in Duchenne muscular dystrophy. *Cochrane Database Syst Rev.* 2015;10:CD005375.

Collis FP, Ponseti (1969). Long-term follow-up of patients with idiopathic scoliosis not treated surgically. *J Bone Joint Surg* 51-A:425–445.

Dangerfield, P.H. (2003). Klassifikation von Wirbelsäulendeformitäten. In: H.R. Weiss: Wirbelsäulendeformitäten. Konservatives Management. München, Pflaum: 78-83.

Daniel KL Cheuk, Virginia Wong, Elizabeth Wraige, Peter Baxter, Ashley Cole (2013). Surgery for scoliosis in Duchenne muscular dystrophy. Editorial Group: Cochrane Neuromuscular Disease Group. Published Online: 28 FEB 2013. Assessed as up-to-date: 31 JUL 2012.

Danielsson AJ, Nachemson AL (2001). Radiologic Findings and Curve Progression 22 Years After Treatment for Adolescent Idiopathic Scoliosis. *Spine* 26 (5):516-552.

Danielsson AJ, Wiklund I, Pehrsson K, Nachemson AL (2001). Health-related quality of life in patients with adolescent idiopathic scoliosis: a matched follow-up at least 20 years after treatment with brace or surgery. *Eur Spine J* 10:278-288.

Eger T, Cordes U (1992). Skoliose – Indikation für ein Sportverbot? *Orthop Praxis* 28: 84-86.

Ferraro C, Masiero S, Venturin A, Pigatto M, Migliorino N (1998). Effect of exercise therapy on mild idiopathic scoliosis. Preliminary results. *Europa Medicophysica*, Vol. 34, No. 1:25-31.

Feskanich D, Willett WC, Stampfer MJ, Colditz, GA (1997). Milk, dietary calcium, and bone fractures in women: a 12-year prospective study. In: *Am J Public Health.* Jun 87(6):992-997.

Flaws B, Wolfe HL (1995). Das Yin und das Yang der Ernährung. Das Handbuch der chinesischen Ernährungslehre. 3rd ed., Scherz Verlag Bern, München, Wien.

Freidel K, Petermann F, Reichel D (1999). Stationäre Intensivrehabilitation bei Skoliose. Medizinischer und psychosozialer Outcome. VZR, Bremen

Glassman SD, Bridwell K, Dimar JR, Horton W, Berven S, Schwab F. (2005). The impact of positive sagittal balance in adult spinal deformity. *Spine* 30(18):2024-9.

Grivas TH, Vasiliadis E, Chatziargiropoulos TH, Polyzois VD, Gatos K. (2003). The effect of a modified Boston brace with anti-rotatory blades on the progression of curves in idiopathic scoliosis: aetiologic implications. *Pediatric Rehabilitation* 6(2-3): 237-242.

Güth V, Abbink S, Götze HG et al. (1976). Kinesiologische und elektromyographische Untersuchungen über die Wirkung des Milwaukee-Korsetts. *Z. Orthop* 114: 480–486.

Güth V, Abbink S, Götze HG (1978). Ganguntersuchungen an Patienten mit idiopathischen Skoliosen und der Einfluß des Milwaukee-Korsetts auf das Gangbild. *Z. Orthop* 116:631–640.

Hagena Ch, Hagena Ch (1997). Konstitution und Bipolarität: Erfahrungen mit einer neuen Typenlehre. 2. Aufl., Haug, Heidelberg.

Hawes M. (2006). Impact of spine surgery on signs and symptoms of spinal deformity. *Pediatr Rehabil.* Oct-Dec; 9(4):318–39.

Howell FR, Mahood JK, Dickson RA (1992). Growth Beyond Skeletal Maturity. *Spine* 17:437–440.

Klisic P, Nikolic Z, Filipovic M u.a. (1991). Krankengymnastik in der Behandlung der leichten Skoliose. In: HR Weiss (Hrsg): Wirbelsäulendeformitäten, *Springer*, Band 1, 1–5.

Landauer F., Wimmer C., Behensky H. (2003). Estimating the final outcome of brace treatment for idiopathic thoracic scoliosis at 6-month follow-up., *Pediatric Rehabilitation* Vol. 6, NO. 3, 1–7.

Landauer F., Wimmer C. (2003). Therapieziel der Korsettbehandlung bei idiopathischer Adoleszentenskoliose. *MOT*, Vol 3, 33–37.

Lehnert-Schroth, CH. (2000). Dreidimensionale Skoliosebehandlung. 6th edition, Urban/Fischer, München.

Lonstein, JE, Carlson JM (1984). The prediction of Curve Progression in untreated idiopathic scoliosis during growth, *J. Bone Joint Surg*, 66-A, 1061–1071.

Mollon G, Rodot JC (1986). Scolioses structurales mineures et kinesithérapie. Etude statistique comparative des résultats. Kinésithér. *Scient* 233:47–56.

Monticone M, Ambrosini E, Cazzaniga D, Rocca B, Ferrante S. Active self-correction and task-oriented exercises reduce spinal deformity and improve quality of life in subjects with mild adolescent idiopathic scoliosis. Results of a randomised controlled trial. *Eur Spine J.* 2014;23(6):1204-14.

Mueller FJ, Gluch H (2012). Cotrel-dubousset instrumentation for the correction of adolescent idiopathic scoliosis. Long-term results with an unexpected high revision rate. *Scoliosis.* 7(1):13. doi: 10.1186/1748-7161-7-13.

Nachemson AL (1968). A long-term follow-up study of non-treated scoliosis. *Acta Orthop Scand* 39: 446.

Nachemson AL (1993). Bracing and Harrington Rod Fusion for Adolescent Idiopathic Scoliosis, are they Outmoded Treatment Methods? Guest Lecture anlässlich des *Ninth International Phillip Zorab Scoliosis Symposiums*, 16–17 September 1993, Cambridge.

Nachemson AL (1993). Psychosocial Factors in Scoliosis. Guest Lecture anlässlich des *Ninth International Phillip Zorab Scoliosis Symposiums*, 16–17 September 1993, Cambridge.

Nachemson AL, Peterson LE (1993). Scoliosis Research Society Brace Study Report, Part I: Effectiveness of Brace Treatment in Moderate Adolescent Idiopathic Scoliosis. *Proceedings of the Scoliosis Research Society Meeting*, 19–23 September, Dublin.

Nachemson, A. L., Peterson, L. E. and Members of Brace Study Group of the Scoliosis Research Society (1995). Effectiveness of treatment with a brace in girls who have adolescent idiopathic scoliosis. *J. Bone Joint Surg.*, 77: 815–822.

Negrini S., Antonini, Gl, Carabalona, R., Minozzi, S. (2003). Physical exercises as a treatment for adolescent idiopathic scoliosis. A systematic review. *Pediatric Rehabilitation* 6: 227–235.

O'leary PT, Sturm PF, Hammerberg KW, Lubicky JP, Mardjetko SM (2011). Convex hemiepiphysiodesis: the limits of vertebral stapling. *Spine* (Phila Pa 1976). Sep 1;36(19):1579-83.

Pauschert R, Niethard F (1994). Ergebnisse der krankengymnastischen Behandlung auf neurophysiologischer Grundlage bei idiopathischer Skoliose: Eine prospektive Analyse. In: HR Weiss (Hrsg): Wirbelsäulendeformitäten. Bd. 3, *Springer* 47–51.

Pehrsson K, Larsson S, Oden A et al. (1992). Long-Term Follow-up of Patients with Untreated Scoliosis. A Study of Mortality, Causes of Death, and Symptoms. *Spine* 17:1091–1096.

Perdriolle R (1992). Natürlicher Verlauf und Prognose der thorakalen und thorakolumbalen idiopathischen Skoliose. In: Weiss HR (Hrsg): Wirbelsäulendeformitäten Bd. 2, Fischer, Stuttgart, Jena, New York, pp 83–84.

Petridou E, Karpathios T, Dessypris N, Simou E, Trichopoulos D (1997). The role of dairy products and nonalcoholic beverages in bone fractures among schoolage children. In: *Scand J Soc Med.*, Jun 25(2):119–125.

Pivetta S (1996). Pregnancy and Scoliosis. In: *Scoliosis, State of the art. Book of Abstracts*, Barcelona 28–30 November.

Pollmer U (1997). Krank durch „gesunde Ernährung": Gesundheitsrisiken durch Getreide und Milch. Vortrag auf dem XII. *Internationalem Symposium für Umweltmedizin*. Bad Ems, 5.–7. September.

Pugacheva N. (2012). Corrective exercises in multimodality therapy of idiopathic scoliosis in children - analysis of six weeks efficiency - pilot study. *Stud Health Technol Inform.* 2012;176:365-71.

Rahmouni A (2002). Skoliose – Der Herausforderung richtig begegnen: Die conservative Behandlung der Skoliose mit der derotierenden Rumpforthese nach Rahmouni. Rahmouni Orthopädietechnik GmbH, Selbstverlag.

Rigo M, Quera-Salva N, Puigdevall N (1991). Effect of the exclusive employment of physiotherapy in patients with idiopathic scoliosis. Retrospective study. In: *Proceedings of the 11th International Congress of the World Confederation For Physical Therapy*. London, 28 July – 2 August: 1319–1321.

Rigo, M. (1999). 3D Correction of Trunk Deformity in Patients with Idiopathic Scoliosis Using Chêneau Brace. In: I.A.F., Stokes (editor). Research into Spinal Deformities 2. (Amsterdam: IOS Press), pp. 362–365.

Rigo M, Reiter CH, Weiss HR (2003). Effect of conservative management on the prevalence of surgery in patients with adolescent idiopathic scoliosis. *Pediatric Rehabilitation*. Jul-Dec;6(3-4):209-14.

Rigo M, Weiss HR (2003). Korsettversorgungsstrategien in der Skoliosebehandlung; in: Weiss HR (Hg.) Wirbelsäulendeformitäten – konservatives Management. Pflaum Verlag, München.

Rigo, M. (2004). Intraobserver reliability of a new classification correlating with brace treatment. *Pediatric Rehabilitation* 7:63.

Ringe JD (Hrg) (1991). Osteoporose. Pathogenese, Diagnostik, Therapiemöglichkeiten. Walter de Gruyter, Berlin, New York.

Romano M, Minozzi S, Bettany-Saltikov J, Zaina F, Chockalingam N, Kotwicki T, et al. Exercises for adolescent idiopathic scoliosis. *Cochrane Database Syst Rev.* 2012;8.

Rowe DE et al. (1997). A meta-analysis of the efficacy of non-operative treatment for idiopathic scoliosis. *J Bone Joint Surg* 79-A, 664–674.

Runow KD (1997). Neue diagnostische Möglichkeiten bei Multipler Chemikalien Sensibilität (MCS) und Chronischem Erschöpfungssyndrom (CFS): Umweltchemikalien, Zahnmetalle, Nahrungsallergene und Pilze. *Vortrag auf dem XII. Internationalem Symposium für Umweltmedizin*, Bad Ems, 5.–7, September.

Schreiber S, Parent EC, Moez EK, Hedden DM, Hill D, Moreau MJ, et al. The effect of Schroth exercises added to the standard of care on the quality of life and muscle endurance in adolescents with idiopathic scoliosis-an assessor and statistician blinded randomized controlled trial: "SOSORT 2015 Award Winner". *Scoliosis* 2015; 10:24.

Stokes, J. (2003). Die Biomechanik des Rumpfes. In: H.R. Weiss: Wirbelsäulendeformitäten. Konservatives Management. München, Pflaum: 59–77.

Temelie B (1995). Ernährung nach den 5 Elementen, Joy Verlag.

Trobisch P, Suess O, Schwab F (2010). Idiopathic Scoliosis. *Dtsch Arztebl Int*; 107(49): 875–84. DOI: 10.3238/arztebl.2010.0875.

van Loon PJ, Kühbauch BA, Thunnissen FB (2008). Forced lordosis on the thoracolumbar junction can correct coronal plane deformity in adolescents with double major curve pattern idiopathic scoliosis. *Spine.* Apr 1;33(7):797–801.

Ward WT RJ, Friel N, Kenkre TS, Brooks MM. SRS 22r Scores in Non-Operated AIS Patients with Curves ≥ 40°. *Proceedings of the 50th Annual Meeting Minneapolis, Minnesota, US, 2015*, September 30th – October 3rd. 2015.

Weinstein SL (1985). Adolescent idiopathic scoliosis: prevalence, natural history, treatment indications. University of Iowa Printing Service, Iowa.

Weinstein, S.L. (1999). Natural history. *Spine*, 24: 2592-2600.

Weiss, HR (1991). The Effect of an Exercise Program on Vital Capacity and Rib Mobility in Patients with Idiopathic Scoliosis. *Spine* 16:88-93.

Weiss HR (1991). Elektromyographsiche Untersuchungen zur skolisosespezifischen Haltungsschulung. *Z Krankengymnastik* 43:1-6.

Weiss HR, Cherdron J (1991). Ergebnisse einer Befragung von Skoliosepatienten nach der Beschwerdeliste von v. Zerssen. *Krankengymnastik* 43:358-360.

Weiss HR, Minnick P (1991). The restrictive ventilation disorders of scoliosis patients under the influence of a physiotherapy rehabilitation program. *Vortrag auf dem 11. Internationalen Kongress der „World Confederation for Physical Therapy"*, London, 28 July – 2 August 1991.

Weiss HR, Cherdron J (1992). Befindlichkeitsänderungen bei Skoliosepatienten in der stationären krankengymnastischen Rehabilitation. *Orthop Prax* 28:87-90.

Weiss HR (1993). Scoliosis-Related Pain in Adults – Treatment Influences. *European Journal of Physical Medicine and Rehabilitation* Vol 3, No 3.

Weiss HR (1994). Zur Anschulung von Orthesen in der Skoliosebehandlung. *Orthopädie Technik* 11.

Weiss HR, Cherdron J (1994). Einflüsse des SCHROTH'schen Rehabilitationsprogramms auf Selbstkonzepte von Skoliosepatienten. *Die Rehabilitation* 33:31-33.

Weiss HR, El Obeidi N (1994). Die Wiederholbarkeit der Bestimmung der Winkelgrade nach Cobb. Vortrag auf dem 4. *Skoliose-Workshop*, April 1994, Sobernheim.

Weiss HR (1995). Möglichkeiten zur Beeinflussung der Sagittalkonfiguration bei idiopathischer Skoliose durch Krankengymnastik. *Orthop Praxis* 31:380-382.

Weiss HR (1995). Standard der Orthesenversorgung in der Skoliosebehandlung. *Med Ortho Tech* 115: 323-330.

Weiss HR (1995). Zur Wertigkeit der muskulären Dysbalance in der Behandlung der idiopathischen Skoliose. *Orthop Praxis* 31:383-387.

Weiss HR (1996). Skoliosebehandlung mit dem „Überkorrekturkorsett" –

Bedeutung des primären Korrektureffekts für das Endresultat. KG 48:199-211.

Weiss HR, Bickert W (1996). Veränderungen elektrokardiographisch objektivierbarer Gesichtspunkte der Rechtsherzbelastung erwachsener Skoliosepatienten durch das stationäre Rehabilitationsprogramm nach SCHROTH. *Orthop Praxis* 32:450-453.

Weiss HR, El Obeidi N, Lohschmidt K, Thomas U (1996). Die stationäre Skolioserehabilitation – eine „Worst-case"-Analyse. *Orthop Praxis* 32:96-100.

Weiss HR, Lohschmidt K, El-Obeidi N, Verres Ch (1997). Preliminary results and worstcase analysis of in-patient scoliosis rehabilitation. *Pediatric Rehabilitation*, 1: 35-40.

Weiss HR (1998). Die aktuelle krankengymnastische Behandlung der Skoliose. *Orthop Praxis* 34:590-597.

Weiss HR, Verres Ch, Lohschmidt K, El Obeidi N (1998). Qualitätssicherung in der stationären Skolioserehabilitation durch vergleichenden Einsatz der automatisierten Oberflächenvermessung. *Orthop Praxis* 34: 450-455.

Weiss HR, Verres Ch, Lohschmidt K, El Obeidi N (1998). Schmerz und Skoliose – besteht ein Zusammenhang? *Orthop Praxis* 34: 602-606.

Weiss HR, Verres Ch, Neumann A (1998). Skoliose und Psyche – Eine Studie bei Jugendlichen und jungen Erwachsenen. *Orthop. Praxis* 34: 367-372.

Weiss HR (1999). Stationäre Rehabilitation bei orthopädischen Erkrankungen. In: F. Petermann und P. Warschburger: Kinderrehabilitation. Hogrefe: 223-232.

Weiss HR, Rigo M, Chêneau J (2000). Praxis der Chêneau Korsettversorgung in der Skoliosetherapie. Thieme, Stuttgart.

Weiss HR (2003). Wirbelsäulendeformitäten – Konservatives Management, Pflaum Verlag, München.

Weiss HR, El Obeidi N, Botens-Helmus CH (2003). Qualitätskontrolle korrigierender Rumpforthesen in der Skoliosebehandlung, *MOT*.

Weiss HR, Weiss G, Schaar HJ (2003). Incidence of surgery in conservatively treated patients with scoliosis. *Pediatr. Rehabil*, 6: 111-118.

Weiss H.R., Weiss G., Petermann F. (2003). Incidence of curvature progression in idiopathic scoliosis patients treated with scoliosis in-patient rehabilitation (SIR): an age- and sexmatched cotrolled study. *Pediatr. Rehabil.* Jan–Mar; 6(1): 23–30.

Weiss HR (2005). Das "Sagittal Realignment Brace" (physio-logic® brace) in der Behandlung von erwachsenen Skoliosepatienten mit chronifiziertem Rückenschmerz (*MOT* 2005; 125: 45–54).

Weiss HR (2007). Differentialindikation der Rumpforthesen in der Skoliosebehandlung, *MOT* 127.

Weiss HR, Werkmann M, Stephan C (2007). Correction effects of the ScoliOlogiC® „Chêneau light" brace in patients with scoliosis, *Scoliosis* 2:2.

Weiss H.R. (Germany), M. Rigo (Spain), T. Kotwitcki (Poland), M. Hawes (USA), F. Landauer (Austria), Boeni, TH, (Switzerland), T.B. Grivas (Greece), T. Maruyama (Japan). Guideline: Indications for Conservative Management of Scoliosis. SOSORT (International Society on Spinal Orthopedic and Rehabilitation treatment) constitutional meeting in Milano, January 2005.

Weiss HR, Goodall D (2008). Rate of complications in scoliosis surgery - a systematic review of the Pub Med literature. *Scoliosis*. Aug 5;3:9.

Weiss HR, Goodall D (2008). The treatment of adolescent idiopathic scoliosis (AIS) according to present evidence. A systematic review. *Eur J Phys Rehabil Med.* 44(2):177-93.

Weiss HR, Bess S, Wong MS, Patel V, Goodall D, Burger E. (2008). Adolescent idiopathic scoliosis - to operate or not? A debate article. *Patient Saf Surg.* Sep 30;2(1):25.

Weiss HR, Seibel S (2010). Scoliosis Short-Term Rehabilitation (SSTR) – A Pilot Investigation, *The Internet Journal of Rehabilitation.* 1: 1.11.

Weiss HR (2011). Treatment was uncritically reported. Dtsch Arztebl Int 108: 11. 189; author reply 189–189; author reply 190 Mar http://www.aerzteblatt.de/v4/archiv/artikel.asp?id=81308

Weiss HR (2011). Befundgerechte Physiotherapie bei Skoliose, 3rd ed., Pflaum Verlag.

Weiss HR, Moramarco M. (2013). Remodelling of trunk and backshape deformities in patients with scoliosis using standardized asymmetric computer-aided design/computer-aided manufacturing braces. *Hard Tissue* 2013 Feb 26;2(2):14.

Weiss HR, Moramarco M (2013). Scoliosis – treatment indications according to current evidence. *OA Musculoskeletal Medicine.* Mar 01;1(1):1.

Weiss HR, Moramarco M, Moramarco K. (2013). Risks and long-term complications of adolescent idiopathic scoliosis surgery vs. non-surgical and natural history outcomes. *Hard Tissue.* Apr 30;2(3):27.

Weiss HR, Seibel S (2013). Region of Interest (ROI) in the radiological follow-up of patients with scoliosis. *Hard Tissue*, June 1; 2(4):33.

Weiss HR, Turnbull D, Tournavitis N, Borysov M (2016) Treatment of Scoliosis- Evidence and Management (Review of the Literature). *Middle East J Rehabil Health.* 2016;3: epub ahead of print 2. April.

Weiss HR, Karavidas N, Moramarco M, Moramarco K: Long-term effects of untreated Adolescent Idiopathic Scoliosis – Review of the literature. *Asian Spine Journal*, in press.

Werle J (Hrg.) (1995). Osteoporose und Bewegung. Springer, Berlin.

Westrick E, Ward W. Adolescent idiopathic scoliosis: 5-year to 20-year evidence-based surgical results. *J Pediatr Orthop.* 2011;31(1 Suppl):S61 - S8.

Wicharz J (1991). Besser leben trotz Osteoporose. Echo-Verlag, Köln.

Winter, R.B. (1995). Classification and Terminology. In: Moe's Textbook of Scoliosis and Other Spinal Deformities, Philadelphia Saunders, pp 39–43.

Ziegler R (1990). Was ist gesichert in der Therapie der Osteoporose? *Internist* 31: 680–688.

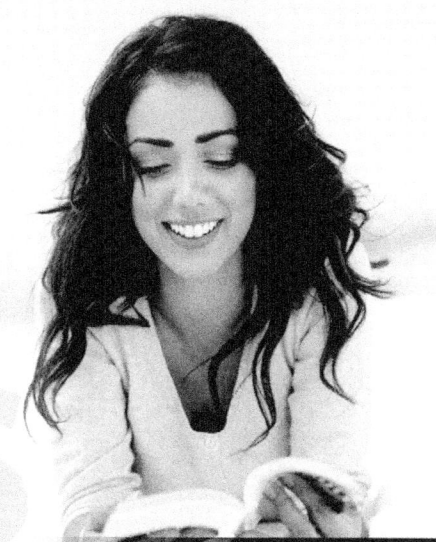

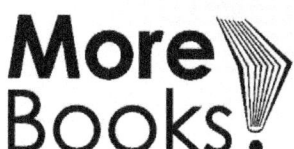

I want morebooks!

Buy your books fast and straightforward online - at one of the world's fastest growing online book stores! Environmentally sound due to Print-on-Demand technologies.

Buy your books online at
www.get-morebooks.com

Kaufen Sie Ihre Bücher schnell und unkompliziert online – auf einer der am schnellsten wachsenden Buchhandelsplattformen weltweit!
Dank Print-On-Demand umwelt- und ressourcenschonend produziert.

Bücher schneller online kaufen
www.morebooks.de

OmniScriptum Marketing DEU GmbH
Bahnhofstr. 28
D - 66111 Saarbrücken   info@omniscriptum.com
Telefax: +49 681 93 81 567-9   www.omniscriptum.com

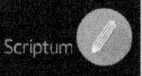

Printed in Great Britain
by Amazon